RUBBER BAND

TAMILEE WEBB'S ORIGINAL

WORKOUT

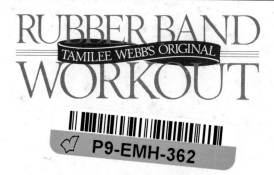

RUBBER BAND

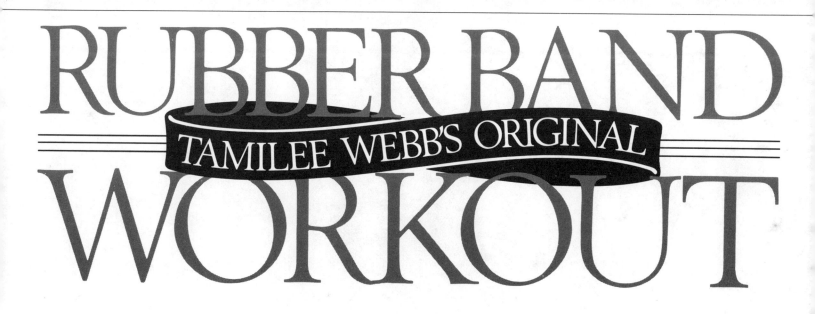

TAMILEE WEBB'S ORIGINAL

WORKOUT

BY TAMILEE WEBB WITH JULIE HOUSTON ● PHOTOGRAPHS BY CHUCK CARLTON

WORKMAN PUBLISHING, NEW YORK

**Library of Congress Cataloging in
Publication Data**

Webb, Tamilee.
    Tamilee Webb's original rubber band workout.
    1. Isotonic exercise. I. Houston, Julie.
II. Carlton, Chuck. III. Title. IV. Title: Original
rubber band workout.
RA781.2.W43 1986   613.7′1   86-11129

ISBN 0-89480-056-6

With the cooperation of Graymont Enterprises, Inc.

Manufactured in the United States of America
First printing August 1986
10 9 8 7 6 5 4 3

Workman Publishing Company, Inc.
1 West 39 Street
New York, New York 10018

With deepest gratitude, this book is
dedicated to Susan Calhoun, Founder
and Director of Fitcamp: Fitness
Instructors Training Camps, for her
support, encouragement and friendship,
and for making The Rubber Band
Workout a part of the Fitcamp program,
where it has been introduced to
thousands of fitness instructors
nationally and internationally.

ACKNOWLEDGMENTS

I would like to thank the following friends, family members and business associates for their support, influence and help:

Ruth Clapper, my manager and friend, who acknowleged my program and helped me to get it published as a book. Millie Glinsky, Fitcamp participant, for informing her sister Sally Kovalchick, of Workman Publishing, that The Rubber Band Workout was no gimmick and really works. The entire Workman staff for their enthusiasm. Julie Houston, my writer, for her speedy and professional work despite our being on opposite coasts.

The Fitcamp staff: Susan Calhoun, Sylvania Reyna, Doug Graham and Teresa Triplett Boyer for teaching, training and inspiring hundreds of other professional fitness instructors to utilize The Rubber Band Workout and many other innovative programs. To these Fitcamp participants, as well as those in the International Dance Exercise Association (IDEA) and the Rubber Band Workshops, I owe much gratitude for keeping an open mind to allow growth, sharing and caring in the programs they offer. Endorsing The Rubber Band Workout as a safe, fun exercise program, they have introduced it to thousands of consumers who look to the professional fitness instructor for guidance in reaching their fitness goals.

In a similar vein, I thank the Golden Door Fitness Staff for presenting The Rubber Band Workout as a Golden Door Special Class, and the guests for their enthusiastic support of this program.

I am indebted to Peter Francis, Ph.D., and Lorna Francis, Ph.D., for their advice and counsel, for their time and knowledge, and for supporting all of us who are working to bring safe, sound education to the expanding field of fitness. They have my highest respect.

I want to thank Dr. Art Ulene for his support and enthusiasm.

A special thanks to a dear friend, Mindy Marinos, for introducing me to my first aerobics class and the exciting world of physical fitness.

For those who have been with me from the start, sharing my belief that The Rubber Band Workout is something everyone could enjoy and that one day this book would become real, I thank Sue Gatlin, Joanne Burger, Kris Alexander, Ronny Schumann and my entire family.

PREFACE

The use of rubber bands as a means of providing resistance for strength training is not a new idea, but Tamilee Webb has elevated the technique to an art form! A number of years ago we had our first opportunity to watch Tamilee teach a rubber band class at a fitness workshop, and we became fascinated by her unique approach to this type of progressive resistance training. Suddenly a familiar and monotonous clinical procedure that we had undergone on linament-soaked athletic training tables had become a dynamic social experience that was fun.

In the past few years Tamilee has relentlessly pursued experts in the field of sports medicine in search of information about the potential benefits and risks of each exercise that she has used. She has directed as much of her energies toward the safety aspects of this workout as she has worked on the creative components that make it universally appealing.

No one has proprietary rights to this wonderful type of training, and so we predict that the success of this book will encourage many others to emulate Tamilee's techniques and her remarkable style. She will be "a tough act to follow"!

Peter R. Francis, Ph.D.
Lorna L. Francis, Ph.D.
San Diego State University

FOREWORD

If you think all exercise programs are alike, you're in for a real surprise. *Tamilee Webb's Original Rubber Band Workout* is different in an important way: it's the first exercise program to use the resistance of rubber bands in a systematic way to tone and strengthen muscles throughout the body.

If you're skeptical about using rubber bands for strength training, you're not alone. I was skeptical, too, when I first heard about it. All doubts were gone soon after I got the chance to "pump rubber." Just five minutes work with the rubber bands convinced me that their resistance is just as real—and just as effective—as the equivalent resistance provided by heavy weights or weight-training machines.

The comparison ends there. Rubber bands are easier to use and, I think, more fun. They are inexpensive and they are portable, so you can keep doing your workout wherever your travels take you.

There's another reason why I'm especially enthusiastic about the *Original Rubber Band Workout:* it meets an important need that is missed by almost all popular exercise programs. Most people assume they can stay fit by doing aerobic exercise, but there's more to it than that. Aerobics will build a healthy heart, but you can't call yourself fit in the *overall* sense unless you also have a good balance of muscular strength and joint flexibility.

Tamilee Webb's *Original Rubber Band Workout* is the perfect complement to any aerobic exercise program. It's a serious toning and strengthening program that has been developed in a thoughtful and deliberate fashion.

Ms. Webb has spent many years developing and perfecting the routines that make up this program. Each one has been carefully thought out to provide you with an enjoyable program that produces results. You can also take comfort from knowing that some of the world's leading exercise experts have reviewed the routines, adding their wisdom and experience to the final product.

I'm delighted to see the *Original Rubber Band Workout* created, and I think you'll feel the same way after you've used it for a while. Make it a regular part of your conditioning program and you'll soon be looking and feeling your very best.

Art Ulene, M.D.
"The Family Doctor"
of NBC's *Today* show

9

CONTENTS

CONTENTS

3 THE RUBBER BAND WORKOUTS: Five Customized Programs for the Beginner to the Very Advanced 109

THE BASIC TEN-STRETCH SEQUENCE

THE FIVE WORKOUTS

INTRODUCTION

I have been interested in fitness all my life. First just for pleasure; then as an educational pursuit, getting a Master's Degree in Physical Education, with strength training and exercise science my specialties; and finally as a career.

I developed The Rubber Band Workout for busy people who find it difficult to incorporate fitness into their lives. As a form of resistance exercise, it is safe, portable (great for travel), easy and lots of fun. The Rubber Band Workout is a strength-training program—without the weights, water or fancy gym equipment. (There are actually five programs to choose from in Part Three, depending on your own level of fitness, lifestyle and how much time you want to invest.) All you need to do the exercises are the rubber bands that come with this book.

As a fitness advisor at the Golden Door Health Spa and Resort in Escondido, California, renowned for its no-nonsense approach to exercise and health, I have introduced The Rubber Band Workout to hundreds of guests who have been delighted with the simplicity and safety of this exercise routine. When I saw that it could strengthen their muscles, improve their appearance and make them feel good all over, I knew it was time to present The Rubber Band Workout to a wider audience. With it, you can achieve the same satisfying results of fitness and conditioning found in the exclusive spas and expensive health clubs—right in your own home, or anywhere you might happen to be with ten minutes extra time!

Tamilee Webb

Tamilee Webb

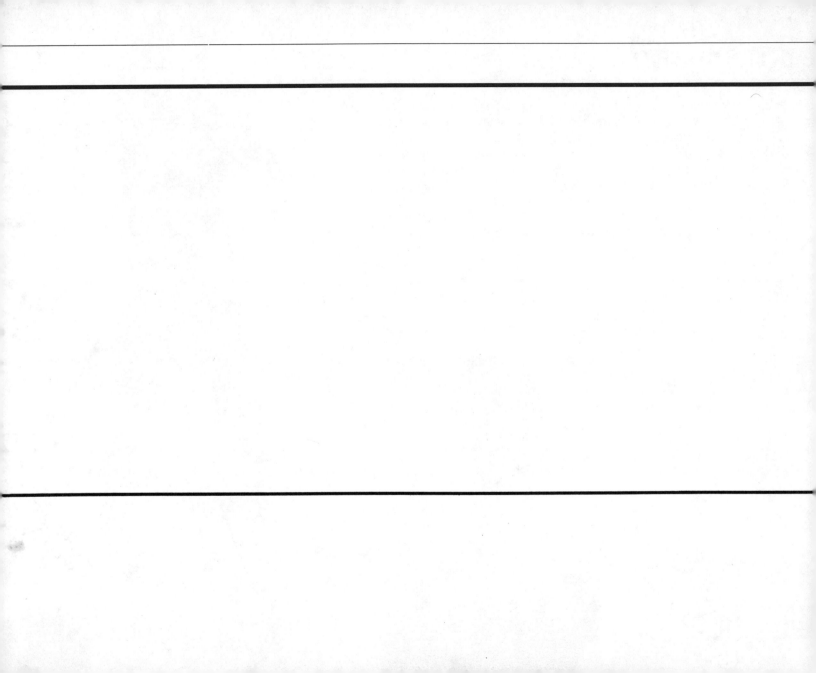

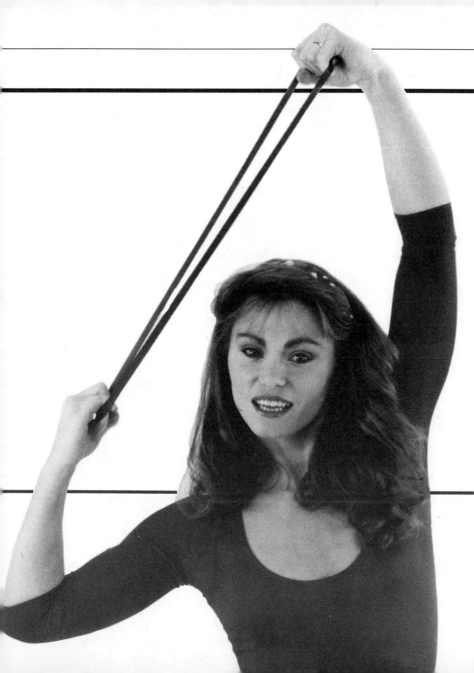

1

INTRODUCING THE RUBBER BAND WORKOUT:

WHAT IT IS AND HOW IT WORKS

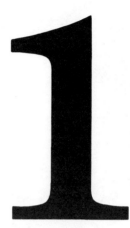

INTRODUCING THE RUBBER BAND WORKOUT

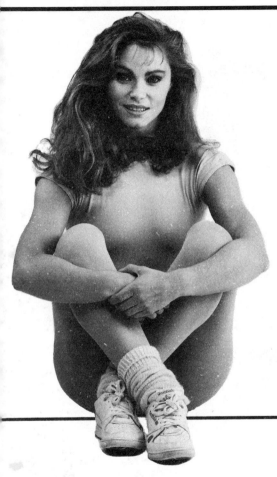

Did you ever think something as simple as pulling on a rubber band could help you look and feel better? Well, it can.

Working the body against the tension of a band is not a gimmick. The concept of working the body with a rubber band was first introduced in sports medicine clinics by physical therapists who were looking for a safe, sure way to help professional athletes recuperate from joint injuries. In physical therapy, the muscles surrounding an injured joint need to be strengthened in order to recover, and resistance exercise with a flexible band—in this case round surgical tubing—provided the perfect means to do this.

Proven effective as a means of rehabilitating sports injuries, exercising with the band soon captured the interest of fitness instructors like myself, who saw its potential as a way to tone, firm and condition the body. Simple to use,

portable and safe, exercising with a band would appeal to anyone—regardless of sex, or level of fitness.

Using readily available flat bands, which are more comfortable for general use than round bands, and choosing exercises that I know can make real improvements in the way the body looks and feels, I created The Rubber Band Workout. Based on the principle of resistance, The Rubber Band Workout is a sound exercise program that will firm, strengthen and condition the major muscles in the body by making them work against the tension of a rubber band.

Resistance exercise is nothing new. It works on the principle that when you overload a muscle, really *make* it work against a force or weight, it will be strengthened. Swimming is a popular form of resistance exercise (moving the body against the resistance of the water). Working with weights is

"You are never too out of shape to incorporate fitness into your life."

INTRODUCING THE RUBBER BAND WORKOUT

resistance exercise (ankle weights, hand weights, the weights in a gym). Using a Nautilus machine, or similar body conditioning equipment, is a form of resistance exercise. Each of these various exercise programs works on the theory that when resistance is utilized, the muscles are pushed to work harder than they would if they were simply moving within their usual capacity.

Our muscles are working against different forms of resistance all the time: the door or window we push open, the groceries we carry home, or the weight of the body itself, lifting our legs to climb stairs or getting ourselves out of bed in the morning. These are everyday "loads of resistance" most of us meet subconsciously. When resistance is increased, however, we feel the effects of the added exertion—a sore back after lugging a heavy suitcase around, or stiff leg muscles after too much walking all at once. Usually, the muscles that are

briefly pushed beyond their capacity quickly settle back to their normal level of inactivity and no longer feel sore.

The few everyday instances when we make our muscles work harder—and the discomforts that may result—make a case for resistance exercise. In our daily routine most of us use only *some* muscles, while other muscles hardly get used at all. A program of resistance exercises helps strengthen *all* the muscles, balancing out the body so it can perform at its peak without risking injury. When resistance exercises are incorporated into a regular fitness program, the muscles become firmer and more efficient, stronger and better conditioned. The whole body benefits— both in its appearance and in how it functions—from the improvements made in the muscle system.

As a form of resistance exercise, The Rubber Band Workout conditions the body without weights, water or fancy

"What is good for one person is not always good for another. Find the exercises that work best for you and use them to your advantage."

INTRODUCING THE RUBBER BAND WORKOUT

gym equipment. Simple as it is, The Rubber Band Workout is as effective as any other resistance exercise, and it is a good deal more fun than many other strengthening programs.

Put the book down for a moment and feel how The Rubber Band Workout uses resistance.

First, hold your arms out straight in front of you and slowly open and close them a few times. Make a mental note of how this feels.

Now, hold the ends of the rubber band in two fists (knuckles facing each other) and do the same exercise.

Can you feel how much harder your muscles had to work when you used the rubber band?

The Rubber Band Workout exercises more than the arms and the upper body. You can put the band around your ankles, knees, thighs (different "points of resistance") to work the front and back thighs, abdomen and buttocks just as

effectively as the front and back of the arms. The *whole* body gets a Rubber Band Workout!

The exercises in the The Rubber Band Workout concentrate on working one muscle or muscle group at a time, applying resistance by first, positioning the band to isolate the muscle (front of arm, front of thigh), and then working that muscle in slow, controlled repetitions against the tension of the band.

Because the band isolates muscles and works them individually, if you concentrate on each exercise as you do it, you will *really feel*—probably for the first time in any exercise routine—those muscles moving as they get the extra benefit of working against the resistance of the rubber band. And you will feel how much more you will be getting out of those movements, because resistance is involved and because the *band* is coaxing your muscles into working harder and

more effectively against that added tension. *You* don't even have to think about it!

THE PUSH-PULL MUSCLE SYSTEM— MUSCLES HAVE PARTNERS

Aware of it or not, all of the muscles in our body form an intricate system of push and pull partners—moving either toward or away from the body as they work against resistance. Think of the muscles as partners, each one part of a two-muscle team. One is a push (extension), the other a pull (flexion), and they compliment each other.

You *pull* a tumbler of water toward your mouth and *push* it back down on the table. You *push* a vacuum across the rug and *pull* it back. With almost every gesture you make, the muscles you use are part of a two-muscle team.

The Rubber Band Workout

concentrates on strengthening both partners in the team to balance out the system. Put your left hand on the front of the right upper arm and curl the right arm up toward your body. Feel the muscle under your hand. That is your biceps working.

Now feel its partner. Put your left hand on the back of the right arm and push the right hand against a table. As you press, feel the muscle in the back of the right arm. That is the triceps working against the resistance of the table.

Do the same with your thighs. Sit down and place one hand on top of your thigh. Straighten the lower leg. That's your very strong quadriceps muscle working! Now place the hand on the back of the same thigh. Cross your ankles to provide resistance, and curl your leg back. Your hamstring muscles are doing the work.

Chest and shoulders, inner thighs and outer thighs, abdomen and lower back— they are all muscle team partners that need to be kept in top form to perform safely.

For some tasks, assisting muscles come into play. If the chest (the push partner to the upper back) needs help pushing a piece of furniture across the room, for example, it calls on other push muscles in the upper body—the shoulders and the back of the arms—to assist with the job. When needed, these assisting muscles will also come into play with some resistance exercises.

While most ordinary tasks require work from both muscle partners, this does not mean they require *equal* work from both. The use of one muscle more than its partner creates an imbalance in the relative increase in strength of the two muscles. This muscle imbalance can cause discomfort and injuries.

"Shin splints" is a good example. This common discomfort in the front of the

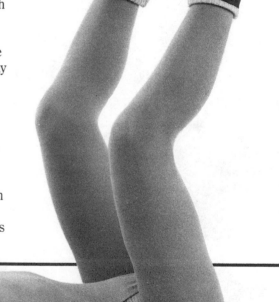

"Fitness should not be pain or punishment, but rather an award that you can wear throughout life."

INTRODUCING TH[E RU]BBER BAND WORKOUT

Shoulder (Deltoids)
PUSH & PULL

Front of Arm (Biceps)
PULL

Chest (Pectoralis major and minor)
PUSH

Hip Flexor (Iliopsoas)
PULL

Stomach (Rectus abdominis)
PULL

Inner Thigh (Adductors)
PULL

Front of Thigh (Quadriceps)
PUSH

Shin (Tibialis anterior)
PULL

shins can occur when the calf muscle in the back of the lower leg becomes so tight that it pulls its weaker, opposing partner in the front of the leg with such force that it can tear the muscle or even damage the shin bone and the connecting tendons. Women who wear high heel shoes tend to experience shin splints because they are always working the calf. To avoid shin splints, the muscles in the front of the leg need to be strengthened and the muscles in the back of the leg need to be stretched.

Back problems are another example of muscle imbalance and the trouble it can cause. Eight out of ten people suffer back injuries because they overuse their backs—carrying heavy objects, or leaning over to pick them up, with the muscles in the lower back bearing the brunt of the load and getting tighter and tighter. We need to stretch out those tight back muscles and take the pressure off the lower back. Moreover, we need to strengthen their opposing partner, the stomach muscles or abdominals.

By strengthening the muscles as partners in The Rubber Band Workout, you can help prevent muscular imbalance, which can cause discomfort and injuries. When they can, we want those weaker muscles to take on some of the responsibility for what needs to get done—to help prevent muscle injury, to help support the load of the stronger partner, to *look* better because they are all toned up.

Each exercise in The Rubber Band Workout deals with a very specific muscle that you will be working. Concentrate on that muscle and how it feels as you perform the exercise. Get to know the muscle you are working and what it wants, and then think about what its *partner* needs and wants. Work both members of the team, strengthening (and stretching) the weaker; stretching (and keeping strong) its too-tight,

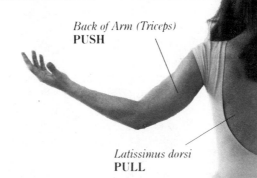

Back of Arm (Triceps)
PUSH

Upper Back (Rhomboids)
PULL

Latissimus dorsi
PULL

Lower Back (Erector spinae)
PULL

*Buttocks
(Gluteus maximus and minimus)*
PUSH & PULL

Outer Thigh (Gluteus medius)
PUSH

Back of Thigh (Hamstrings)
PULL

Calf (Gastrocnemius/Soleus)
PUSH

stronger partner. That's getting the most out of The Rubber Band Workout.

MUSCLE VS. FAT

The Rubber Band Workout cannot accomplish everything you want for your body. It can firm and condition your muscles and it can help you lose inches. But if getting rid of excess fat is one of your objectives, you will need to broaden your fitness program to include aerobics (to burn off the fat) as well as proper eating habits (to keep it off). You can do fifty leg lifts and fifty sit-ups, but if it is *fat* you are trying to eliminate, all your efforts with resistance exercise will go unrewarded. Those lifts and sit-ups are working muscles, not the fat! Do them— but to get rid of the fat, do aerobics, too.

Have you ever tried the little "pinch test" found on the back of the cereal box? It helps determine how much, if any, excess fat there is on the body.

Pinch your stomach. If there's more than an inch of fat between your fingers, you may want to reevaluate your diet and engage in aerobic activity.

Try the pinch test on other areas of your body. Did you notice some areas you pinched were fattier than others? We all store fat in different places on the body—depending, it seems, on heredity. Thus, if your mother had fat legs, and her mother had fat legs, and so on, you may also tend to store more fat in the legs. That does not mean you will definitely have fat legs because others in your family had them. It just means that should you accumulate excess fat, it will probably be stored in your legs and you might have to work a little harder than the next person to keep the excess fat off.

Don't believe the common fallacy that doing exercise will turn fat into muscle. It is impossible! You can decrease the amount of fat in and around the muscle,

condense and condition the muscle and thereby lose inches, but you will never turn fat into muscle as you do it. Conversely, if you stop exercising, you will not turn muscle into fat.

Be clear on what you are doing when you do The Rubber Band Workout. If you are working to get rid of excess fat, the exercises will help you meet your goal, but remember that aerobics and good eating habits are the other half of what you'll need to see results.

Be realistic about the time it will take to get into shape. Naturally, we want to see improvements in our body when we work out and diet. We want everything fast! But nature does not grant us our every wish and getting into shape is a slower, more arduous process for some people than for others. Do not believe that if you start working on those hips and thighs today, by tomorrow the unsightly dimples and bulges will be gone. It just won't happen that quickly.

A Simple Aerobic Exercise: *Before doing this exercise, be sure the chair is sturdy and that it will support your weight. Step up onto the chair—leading with the right foot and bringing the left foot up so that both feet are on the chair (left). Step down, again leading with the right foot and supporting your weight with the left foot (right).*

Maintaining a steady pace, continue stepping up and down for as long as possible, but no more than 15 minutes.

WHAT YOU GET FROM THE RUBBER BAND WORKOUT

The Rubber Band Workout benefits the *whole* body. It can help you:

• Lose inches and look thinner. Dieting may lose pounds, but it doesn't always change the way you look; while *inches,* lost through an exercise program, can make you look thinner. You can lose ten pounds and still wear a size 14 or lose five pounds and wear a size 12.

• Increase strength and energy for sports and fitness activities. The Rubber Band Workout is resistance exercise without weights or other equipment. If you go to the gym, that's great—but when you can't get there, do The Rubber Band Workout.

• Balance out body proportions, regardless of body type. Too many people who diet go from a large pear to a small pear—losing weight but keeping that same bottom-heavy shape. The Rubber Band Workout can help you balance things out so your upper half is more in proportion with your lower half. Individual proportions (for example, short legs) obviously cannot be changed. But with The Rubber Band Workout those same short legs can be reshaped to be stronger, firmer and well defined.

To see and feel improvements, you

"Gradually incorporate fitness into your lifestyle. Set reasonable goals and you won't be disappointed."

should do The Rubber Band Workout two or three times a week, every other day. *Always* give the muscles a day off between workouts to relax (this goes for any kind of resistance exercise). No matter which of the workouts you choose in Part Three, this day off between exercise sessions is important for the well-being of your body.

When you turn to Part Three, you will find several different workouts. One to get in shape. One to stay in shape. One for the times you are sitting. Another to do if you have only ten minutes for exercise. Still another to do when your body is strong and you want more of a challenge. *You* choose the program that fits your lifestyle and schedule. By doing The Rubber Band Workout, you will be giving your body what it needs. And it *needs* fitness. You give it food. You give it time for entertainment. Give it some fitness, too! Make fitness a part of your life.

SAFETY REMINDERS

1. Check the rubber bands before every workout for holes, tears, thinness and overuse, especially around the knot of the double rubber band. Never try to break the rubber band by stretching it beyond a reasonable point.

2. Never pull the rubber band toward the face or toward others around you in case it should break or slip loose. Always look away from the band when using it near the face.

3. Keep the wrists straight so the hand is in line with the forearm.

4. Wear protective garments between the rubber band and the skin—sweatpants, socks, leg warmers, a leotard. If you want to protect the palm, wear a wrist band or the cut-off top of a tube sock around the hand. Always wear shoes.

5. Control the band at all times; it should not control you. Always maintain tension in the band when releasing it back to a starting position.

6. Never jog with the rubber bands around the ankles.

7. Have a complete physical checkup before starting this or any fitness program if you are: a man over 40; a woman over 45; an individual with high blood pressure, arthritis, varicose veins or bursitis; or if you are pregnant. The Rubber Band Workout is *not* intended for children. If you have any questions or concerns regarding your health, consult your physician.

8. Listen to your body. If pain occurs, discontinue that particular exercise and substitute another exercise for that muscle group.

9. Never become relaxed about safety. Whether working out, swimming or driving, be alert. Accidents frequently happen when they are least expected. For happy, healthful fitness, your own safety is a primary concern.

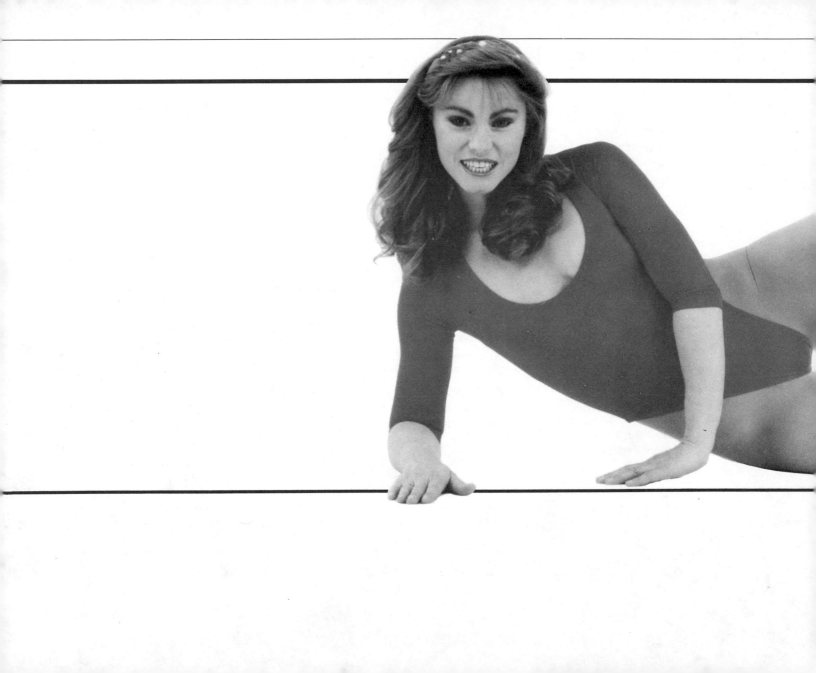

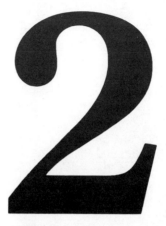

2

THE BASICS OF THE RUBBER BAND WORKOUT:

RESISTANCE EXERCISES AND THE USE AND CARE OF THE BAND

THE BASICS OF THE RUBBER BAND WORKOUT

Now that you know what exercising with a rubber band is all about, it is necessary to master the individual resistance exercises that comprise the workouts that follow this section. Arranged by muscle and muscle group, each exercise concentrates on working one muscle of the push-pull system. Learn all of them so that if you find that an exercise suggested in one of the workouts does not feel right for you, you can substitute another from the selection presented for that muscle group. Altering exercises will also add variety to your workout. But do at least one exercise in each muscle group. That way you will be working both members of the team—strengthening (and stretching) the weaker, and stretching (and keeping strong) its stronger partner—to help balance out the body.

The resistance exercises in this book are done with either a single band or with two bands tied together to make a double band. Your own strength will determine which one is for you. This is an important consideration. You should be comfortable using the band—a band that is too tight for your strength can put stress on the joints.

If you have never worked out with resistance, start the program with the double band. It will be more comfortable to use in the beginning because you will work with less tension (resistance) than with the single band. When using the double band becomes too easy, switch to the single band for more resistance.

For those with longer limbs or a greater range of motion, though, the single band's stretch may not be enough for an effective workout. (Remember, never pull the band past a reasonable point or it could break.) The extra length of the double band will provide enough stretch to accommodate longer limbs. As the band stretches, the resistance increases, so the double band can be suitable for advanced workouts.

HOW THE EXERCISES ARE SET UP

Each exercise is presented so that it can be easily followed by the beginner or advanced. Because the movements of the exercise are the same—whether you use the double band or the single band—it is necessary to show them only once. Therefore, each exercise is presented with two starting positions—one for the beginner using the double band and one for the advanced using the single band. Steps 2 and 3 follow the advanced starting position and show only the single band. If you are a beginner, assume the beginner starting position and continue the exercise with the movements described in steps 2 and 3.

BASIC BAND POSITIONS

You can hold the band either with your fists or with a few fingers, whichever is most comfortable for you. Most people, including myself, prefer the fist grip (the band across the palm and the fingers closed over it), because it seems more secure and less apt to create a burning sensation around the fingers. I've shown and described holding the band this way throughout the book, but try it both ways and see which hand position you like better.

After doubling the bands (see photographs at right), continue to use the fist grip for the double band that's most comfortable for you. You can alter the degree of resistance by changing the position of your grip. For more resistance, grip the double band *on* the knot; for less resistance, grip the double band *below* the knot.

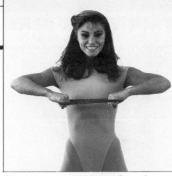

Single band held in two fist grips, palms down and knuckles facing.

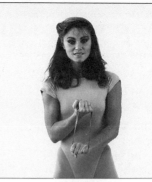

Single band held in two fist grips, right palm up and left palm down.

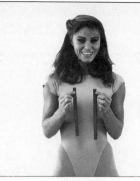

To double the bands:

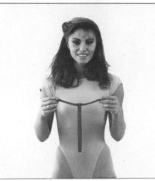

form a T by passing one band through the end of the other band;

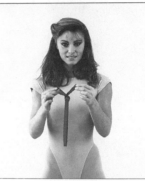

slip the top band through itself around the end of the bottom band to form a knot;

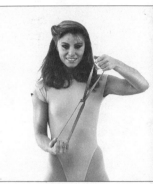

pull the ends of the two loops to tighten the knot.

Double band held on the knot (for more resistance) with the left fist, and the top loop held in a right fist grip, palm up (near right).

Double band held below the knot (for less resistance) with the left fist, and the top loop held in a right fist grip, palm up (far right).

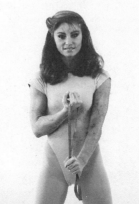

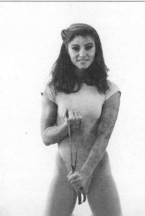

29

THE BASICS OF THE RUBBER BAND WORKOUT

BASIC STANDING POSITION

The basic standing position is always feet flat on the floor, shoulder distance apart; knees slightly bent; shoulders relaxed; stomach pulled in and hips tucked forward. This position gives you a safe, solid base and keeps pressure off the lower back and knees. As you do the standing exercises, periodically check to be sure you maintain the basic position.

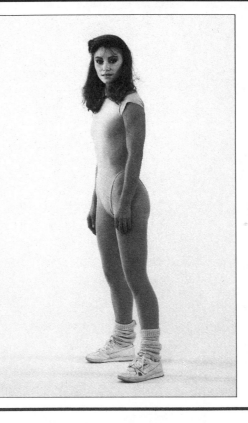

Correct Basic Standing Position.

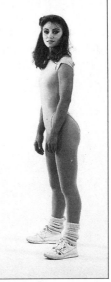

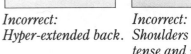

Incorrect: Hyper-extended back.

Incorrect: Shoulders tense and raised.

BASIC SITTING POSITION

Many of the exercises shown in a standing position can also be done sitting in a chair. The basic sitting position is always feet solidly on the ground with knees shoulder distance apart; shoulders relaxed; back straight; stomach pulled in. Any variations on the basic sitting position will be shown with individual exercises. For all, the goal is simply to assume as comfortable a position as you can while working with the band.

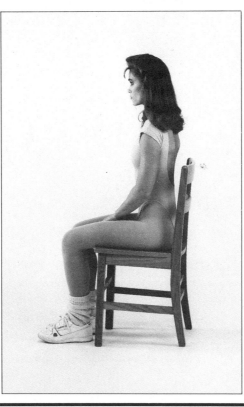

Correct Basic Sitting Position.

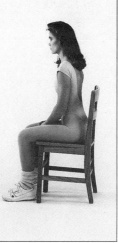

Incorrect: Hyper-extended back.

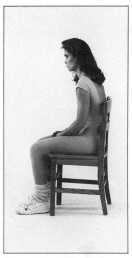

Incorrect: Shoulders forward and back not straight.

THE BASICS OF THE RUBBER BAND WORKOUT

BASIC PRONE POSITION

The most comfortable way to lie face down is with the hips raised slightly to take pressure off the lower back. To do this, place a folded towel or small pillow under the hips. Relax the whole body. Your arms can be straight out or folded under your head; keep your head face down or turn it to one side.

BASIC SUPINE POSITION

The basic supine position is lying flat on your back with legs straight out or with knees bent and feet on the floor. In both instances it is important to keep the lower back flat on the floor by pulling in your stomach muscles and tucking your hips forward. Arms can be straight at the sides or raised over the head.

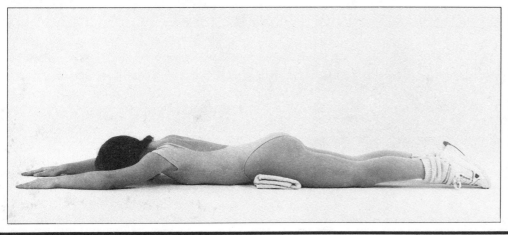

Correct Basic Prone Position.

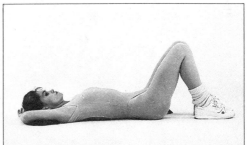

Correct Basic Supine Position.

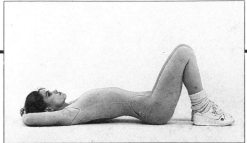

Incorrect: Hyper-extended back.

BASIC FLOOR POSITION, LYING ON ONE SIDE

Many of the leg muscles are worked best when you are lying on your side, but there are several ways to assume this position. It is a matter of which variation is most comfortable for you—propped up on one elbow, lying down on your elbow, or lying all the way down with your arm extended out and your head resting on it.

When you lie on your side, the leg that is closest to the floor is called your base leg. It should be slightly bent to give you a base of support. Your hips and knees should be facing forward. Be sure not to lock the top knee joint.

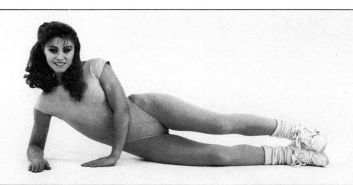

Correct Basic Floor Position, Lying on One Side: propped up on one elbow.

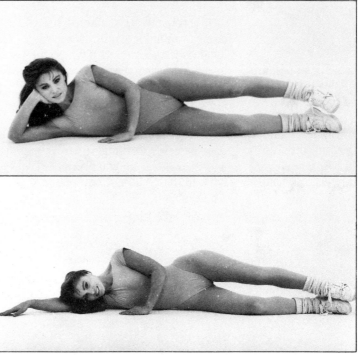

Correct Basic Floor Position, Lying on One Side: lying down on one elbow.

Correct Basic Floor Position, Lying on One Side: lying down with head resting on extended arm.

THE BASICS OF THE RUBBER BAND WORKOUT

BASIC BREATHING PATTERN FOR THE EXERCISES

Many people concentrate so hard when they do an exercise that they forget to breathe and just hold their breath. Your body needs a regular flow of oxygen in order to relax during your stretches and your workout. If you hold your breath, you will tense up.

Try to exhale when you pull the band open (the hard part) and inhale when you release it (the easier part). Breathe evenly.

BAND SAFETY

The bands that come with this book are from SPRI Products (see page 139 for source information) and have been researched and tested by B.F. Goodrich for use in this program. I recommend the SPRI bands because they are durable and safe. If they should break while you exercise with them, they will not snap as forcefully as ordinary bands.

Always check your bands before you use them. Hold them out and look at them carefully to see if they have any small rips, holes or tears. Stretch them to be sure they are not getting thin. If you see any signs of wear, discard them and order new bands.

As an extra measure of safety, always look away from the rubber band when you hold it close to your head in case you lose your grip or the band snaps or breaks.

If you really *think* about what you are doing, you'll do it right. *Always* keep the band under your control when you use it in the exercises. Every move you make should be deliberate; all your concentration should be focused on stretching the band slowly open, and releasing it slowly back in. You will feel your muscles working on both the pull and the release as you bring the band back to the point just before slack. There should always be tension in the band, and you should always be in control of that tension. Never let the band pull you back with it!

SKIN PROTECTION

One of the advantages of The Rubber Band Workout is that it can be done anywhere, anytime—whenever you set aside time from the routine of your day. Almost any loose, comfortable clothes will do, but be sure to put a layer of clothing between your skin and the band for protection: socks or sweats to protect the ankles; pants or tights to protect the calves, knees and thighs. This will prevent skin irritation and pulling on any body hair. Wrist bands worn around your hands prevent the band from slipping and reduce the possibility of discomfort.

Before learning the resistance exercises, study the hand grips and be sure to get comfortable with the four basic positions used in the exercises.

RUBBER BAND WORKOUT TERMS

Base leg: The leg that is closest to the floor or the leg that is holding you up during an exercise.

Before slack: The band's release position in an exercise repetition, just before it loses tension.

Flexibility: The range of motion in a single joint or series of joints.

Locking a joint means holding it stiff. A locked joint can experience stress. Don't lock joints.

Point of resistance: The part of the body where resistance originates. If you hold the band against your waist, for example, the waist is the point of resistance. Or if you place the band around your ankles for outer thigh lifts, the base ankle is the point of resistance.

Range of motion: The range of motion describes the area in space you can cover by moving an arm or a leg. For each person the range of motion varies, depending on the flexibility of the joints.

To curl a part of the body means to bend it in toward the center of the body.

To extend a part of the body means to bend it away from the center of the body.

PAIN IS NOT GAIN

An exercise routine should be fun. A few sore muscles are a sign the body is responding to the workout —but the exercises themselves should not hurt. LISTEN TO YOUR BODY. Exercise a muscle until it tires to the point of fatigue, but no further. The muscle is sending you a message to stop, and it's time to move on to another part of the body. You don't have to *keep* working that muscle to get better results—all you will get is a lot of pain.

Front of Arm Curl

The forearm is the only part of the body that moves during this exercise. Elbows stay close to the body as the fist curls up toward the shoulder.

• Beginners, hold the double band below the knot if you feel too much resistance and above the knot if you need more.

• Keep wrists in line with the forearm as you do the repetitions.

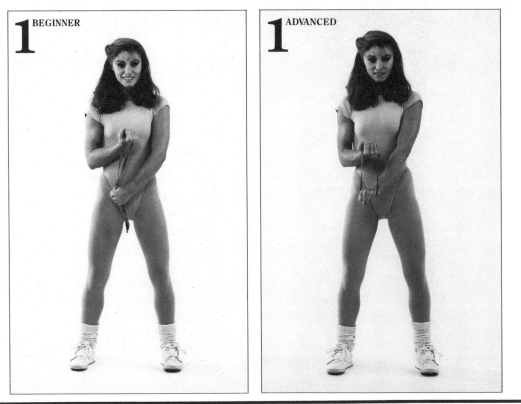

1 BEGINNER

1 ADVANCED

REPETITIONS
Beginner: 8 to 12 for each arm
Advanced: 12 to 16 for each arm

This exercise can also be done in the basic sitting position.

BEGINNER: Basic standing position. Hold the double band below the knot in the left fist, in front of the right hip. Hold the end of the top loop in a right fist grip, palm up and elbows close to the sides. Continue with steps 2 and 3.

ADVANCED: Basic standing position. Hold the single band in two fist grips, right palm up and left palm down. Position the left fist in front of the right hip and the right fist directly above the left fist. Keep elbows close to the sides.

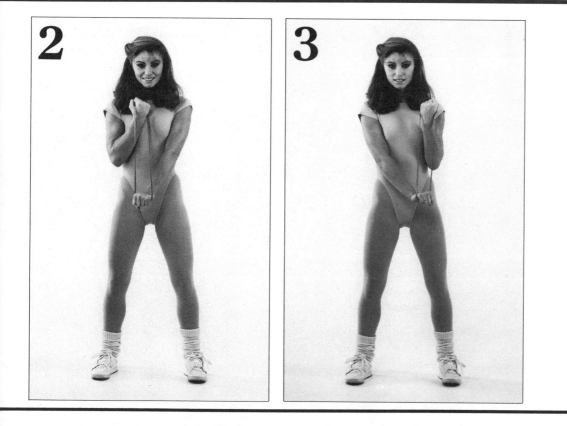

2

3

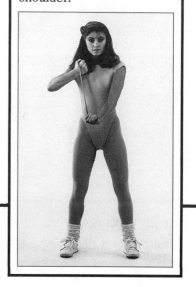

DON'T let the elbow move up and out to the side as you do the repetitions. It must stay close to the body for the front of the arm to benefit from this exercise. Nothing else moves but the forearm, curling up toward the shoulder.

Keep the left hand in position. Curl the right fist toward your right shoulder and slowly release it down to the point before the band goes slack. Curl up and release down, keeping the repetitions smooth, continuous, and controlled.

Reverse hand positions and repeat the exercise with the left arm.

Front of Arm Curl with Foot

The foot is the point of resistance in this exercise. Working the band in a sitting position lessens the tension and is recommended for beginners.

• Do not bend the arm down farther than waist level during the repetitions.

• Keep the working elbow close to the side. The forearm is all that moves during the exercise.

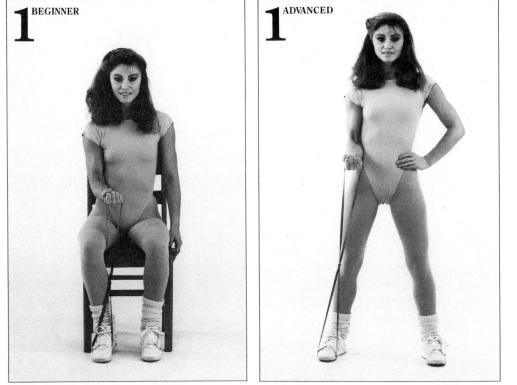

REPETITIONS
Beginner: 8 to 12 for each arm
Advanced: 12 to 16 for each arm

BEGINNER: Basic sitting position. Place one end of the double band around the middle of the right foot, at the arch. Hold the other end of the band in a right fist grip, palm up. Keep the right elbow close to the side. Continue with steps 2 and 3.

ADVANCED: Basic standing position. Place one end of the double band around the middle of the right foot, at the arch. Hold the other end of the band in a right fist grip, palm up. Keep the right elbow close to the side.

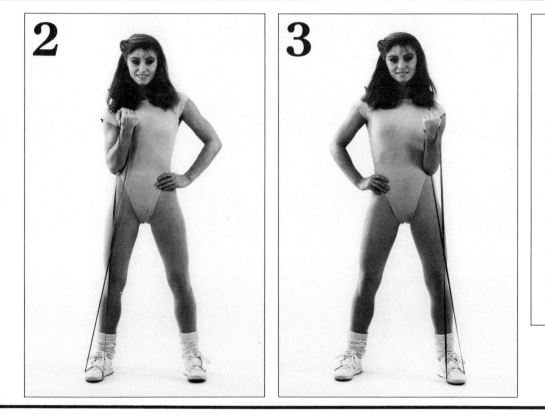

THE BICEPS muscle runs from the inner elbow to the front of the shoulder. This is the muscle that feeds us. It moves the arm in toward the body, toward the mouth or the chest. Its partner, or opposing muscle, is the back of the arm, or triceps. When working the front of the arm, the elbow must be kept next to the body as the forearm curls up. If the elbow moves out, or forward, from this position, the muscles in the shoulder will assist the forearm curl. The front of the arm gets its best workout when it is isolated, or exercised on its own.

Slowly curl the right forearm up toward the shoulder and release it down to waist level. Curl up and release down, keeping the repetitions smooth, continuous, and controlled. Do not let the band snap down below waist level.

Reverse positions and repeat the exercise with the left arm.

Double-Arm Curl

Some people like the idea of working both arms at once the way you might in a weight training room on expensive equipment. It is a good way to vary the exercise for the biceps.

• Keep the elbows close to the side throughout the exercise.

• Do not allow the arms to straighten and the elbow joints to lock.

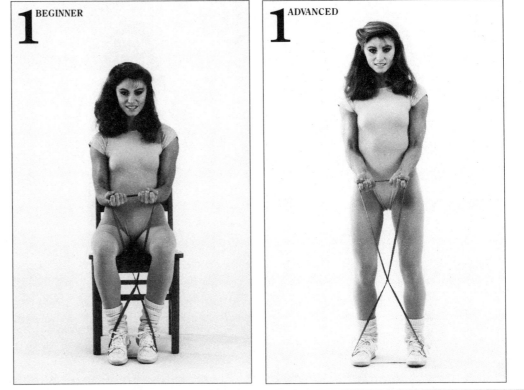

1 BEGINNER

1 ADVANCED

REPETITIONS
Beginner: 8 to 12
Advanced: 12 to 16

BEGINNER: Basic sitting position, with knees apart. Place the feet through one end of the double band, positioning the band under the arches of the feet, and step down on it. Hold the other end of the band in two fist grips, palms up, at waist level. Continue with steps 2 and 3.

ADVANCED: Basic standing position. Place the feet through one end of the double band, positioning the band under the arches of the feet, and step down on it. Hold the other end of the band in two fist grips, palms up, at waist level. Keep the elbows close to the sides.

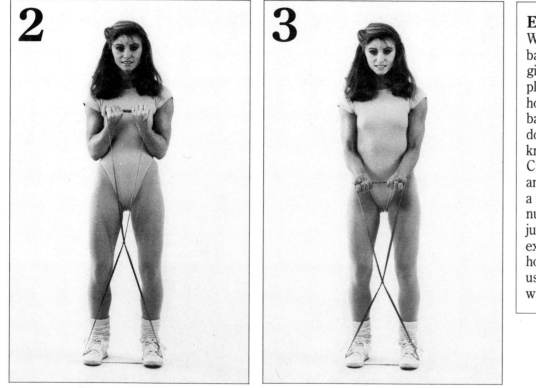

2

3

EXERCISE ON THE GO

When you travel by air, pack the bands in your carry-on luggage and give your biceps a workout on the plane. Settle into your seat and hook each end of the double rubber band around an armrest. Hold the double band on either side of the knot with two fist grips, palms up. Curl the arms up toward the chest and release them down, but only to a point before slack. Do your usual number of repetitions. You'll get just as much out of doing this exercise on a plane as you would at home. There are lots of ways to use the band while traveling—see what you can come up with.

Slowly curl the forearms up toward the chest.

Release the arms down, but do not lock the elbow joint. Curl up and release down, keeping the repetitions smooth, continuous, and controlled.

Back of Arm Press-Down

The back of the arm, or triceps, is usually weaker than its partner, the front of the arm, or biceps. This first exercise for the back of the arm is done by pressing the forearm, or the palm of your hand, down toward the floor. In the exercises that follow, the objective is to tighten up the backs of the arms so they don't wiggle like jelly when you wave goodbye, or sag when you wear a T-shirt or sleeveless dress. In each, the back of the arm gets a workout—the only difference is the direction of the press.

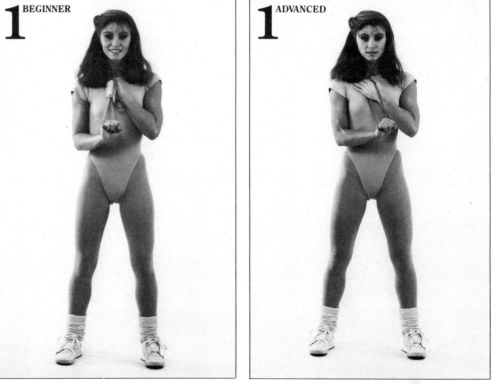

1 BEGINNER

1 ADVANCED

REPETITIONS
Beginner: 8 to 12 for each arm
Advanced: 12 to 16 for each arm

This exercise can also be done in the basic sitting position.

BEGINNER: Basic standing position. Hold the double band on the knot in the left fist, palm in and against the front of the chest. Hold the bottom loop of the band in a right fist grip, palm down. Keep the elbows close to the sides. Continue with steps 2 and 3.

ADVANCED: Basic standing position. Hold one end of the single band against the chest with the left palm. Hold the other end of the band in a right fist grip, palm down. Keep the elbows close to the sides.

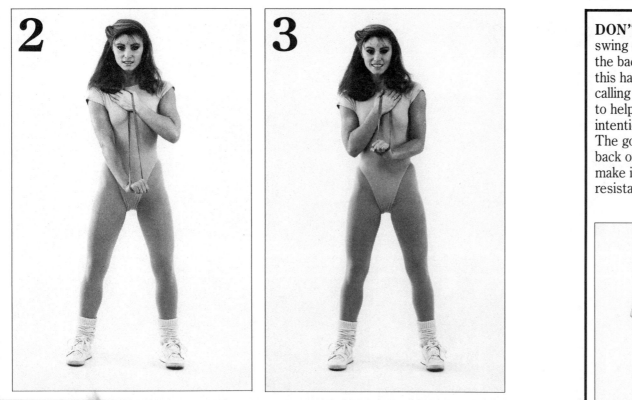

2

3

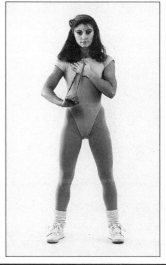

DON'T let the elbow swing out as you work the back of the arm. If this happens, you will be calling on the shoulders to help, which is not the intention of the exercise. The goal is to isolate the back of the arm and make it work against the resistance of the band.

Keep the left hand in position. Press the palm of your right hand down toward the floor. Slowly release the right arm back up to waist level. Press down and release up, keeping the repetitions smooth, continuous, and controlled. Don't let the band snap up.

Reverse hand positions and repeat the exercise with the left arm.

Back of Arm Sideways Press

In this exercise, the shoulder muscle assists but the back of the arm, or triceps, does most of the work. Concentrate on moving only the forearm as you do this exercise. Hold the rest of the arm out at shoulder level with the elbow open to the side.

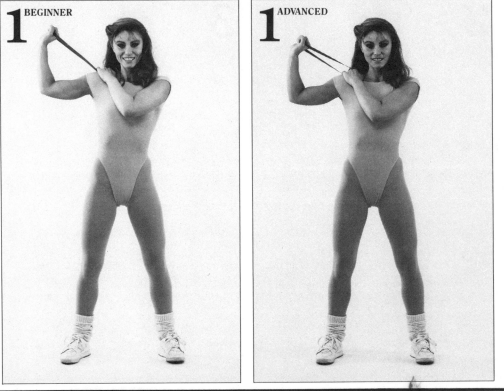

REPETITIONS

Beginner: 8 to 12 for each arm

Advanced: 12 to 16 for each arm

This exercise can also be done in the basic sitting position.

BEGINNER: Basic standing position. Hold the double band at the knot with the left fist and place it on the right shoulder. Hold the end of the top loop in a right fist grip, palm out to the side and wrist in line with the forearm. Continue with steps 2 and 3.

ADVANCED: Basic standing position. Hold one end of the single band on the right shoulder, under the left palm as if you were patting yourself on the shoulder. Hold the other end of the band in a right fist grip, palm out to the side and wrist in line with the forearm.

2

3

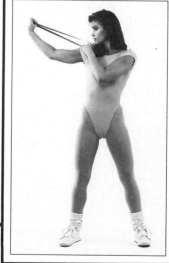

Keep the band in position on your right shoulder. Press the right forearm out to the side. Slowly release the forearm back in without allowing the band to go slack. Press out and release in, keeping the repetitions smooth, continuous, and controlled.

Reverse hand positions and repeat the exercise with the left arm.

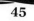

Back of Arm Press-Up

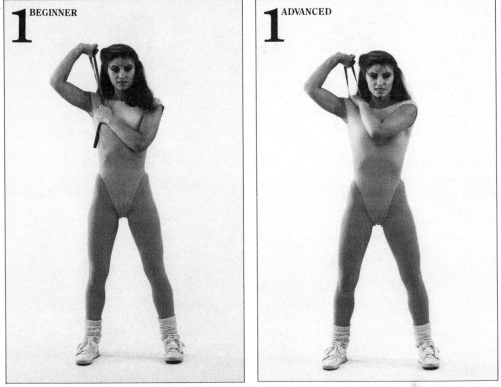

As with the back of arm sideways press, the shoulder muscle assists the triceps to press overhead. Keep the elbow facing out as you do the exercise and move only the forearm.

• Beginners can always hold the double band above the knot to give more resistance or below the knot for less.

• Turn the face away from the band in case it should snap loose.

• Keep the palm extended over the shoulder and the elbow out to the side.

REPETITIONS
Beginner: 8 to 12 for each arm
Advanced: 12 to 16 for each arm

This exercise can also be done in the basic sitting position.

BEGINNER: Basic standing position. Hold the double band at the knot with the left fist and place it at the front of the right shoulder, palm in, at about armpit level. Hold the end of the top loop of the single band in a right fist grip, palm up. Continue with steps 2 and 3.

ADVANCED: Basic standing position. Hold one end of the single band on the right shoulder and under the left palm. Hold the other end of the band in a right fist grip, palm up.

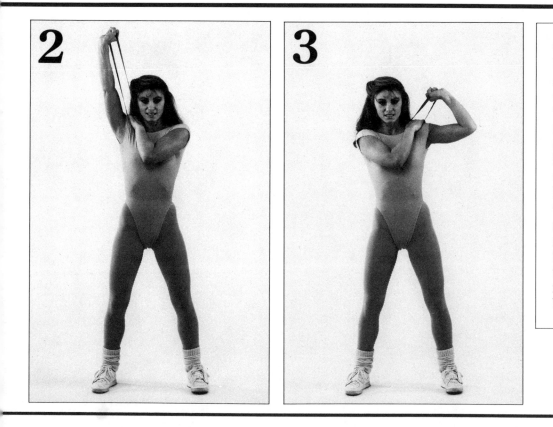

THE TRICEPS muscle runs from behind the elbow to the back of the shoulder. It is the opposing muscle to the front of the arm (biceps). The biceps *pulls* things in toward the body, the triceps *pushes* things away. When we work this muscle, it's always with palms either down or facing away from the body. The back of the arm is usually a lot weaker than the front of the arm, so more exercise variations are given for the back of the arm than the front. When appropriate, keep the elbow next to the side, and really try to isolate and work that back of the arm to firm it up.

Keep the left hand on your right shoulder. Press the right palm up toward the ceiling. Slowly release the arm back down. Press up and release down, keeping the repetitions smooth, continuous, and controlled.

Reverse hand positions and repeat the exercise with the left arm.

Back of Arm Press-Back

Another way to strengthen and firm up the back of the arm is to press against the resistance of the band in a backward motion. Keep the elbow pointed back as you work the arm. Move only the forearm.

• Be sure the wrist remains in line with the forearm.

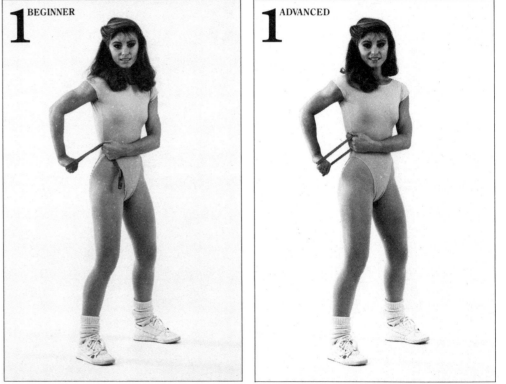

REPETITIONS
Beginner: 8 to 12 for each arm
Advanced: 12 to 16 for each arm

This exercise can also be done in the basic sitting position.

BEGINNER: Basic standing position. Hold the double band at the knot with the left fist, palm in, and place it against the right side at waist level. Hold the end of the top loop in back with a right fist grip, palm facing back, at about hip level. Continue with steps 2 and 3.

ADVANCED: Basic standing position. Hold one end of the single band under the left palm, against the right side of the body at waist level. Hold the other end of the band in a right fist grip, palm facing back, at about hip level.

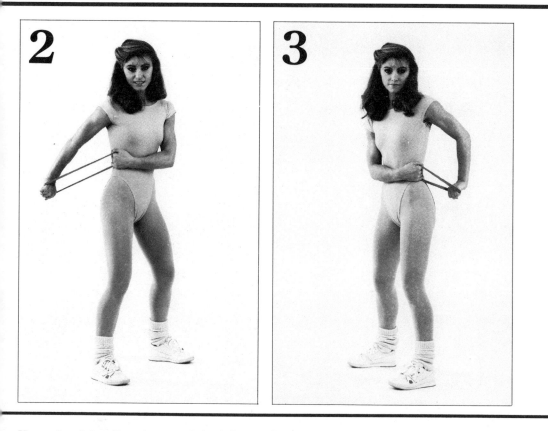

Keep the right elbow bent and the left hand at the waist. Press the right palm straight back as far as possible and slowly release it forward. Press back and release forward, keeping the repetitions smooth, continuous, and controlled.

Reverse hand positions and repeat the exercise with the left arm.

Upper Back Conditioner

At every level of fitness, this basic exercise is safe for the upper back, which tends to be a good deal weaker than its muscle partner, the chest. In addition to strengthening the back, this particular exercise will help prevent the shoulders from hunching, or rounding over—a tendency that increases with inactivity.

• Breathe comfortably as you do the repetitions—exhale as you draw the elbows back, inhale as you release them forward. Keep the shoulders relaxed and the band tensed, and concentrate on working the muscles in the upper back. *Think* about them.

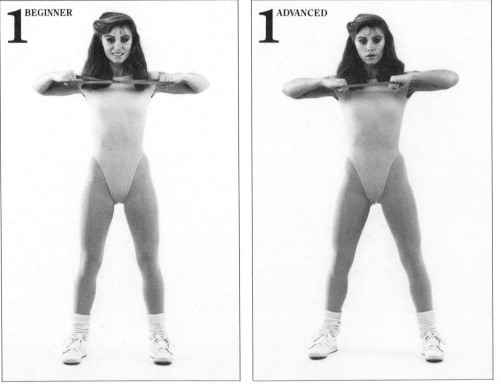

REPETITIONS
Beginner: 8 to 12
Advanced: 12 to 16

This exercise can also be done in the basic sitting position.

BEGINNER: Basic standing position. Hold the double band in two fist grips, palms down, and raise the arms up to shoulder level. Keep the fists close to the body and the elbows up and out to the side. Continue with step 2.

ADVANCED: Basic standing position. Hold the single band in two fist grips, palms down, and raise the arms up to shoulder level. Keep the fists close to the body and the elbows up and out to the side.

2

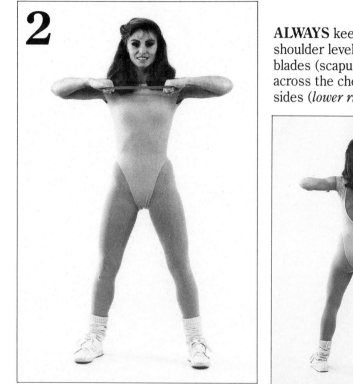

ALWAYS keep the elbows and forearms on the same plane, at shoulder level, and imagine you are squeezing the shoulder blades (scapulae) together (*lower left*). Draw the band straight across the chest, keeping the elbows up and out to the sides (*lower right*).

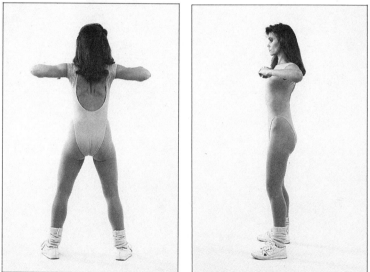

Draw the elbows and shoulders straight back as if you were trying to have the elbows meet behind you. Slowly release the band forward, but don't let the band go slack. Draw back and release forward, keeping the repetitions smooth, continuous, and controlled.

Upper Back Conditioner, Arms Alternating

Correct arm positions are important during this exercise. Keep the wrists in line with the forearms and, as you pull the arm down, keep the elbow out to the side.

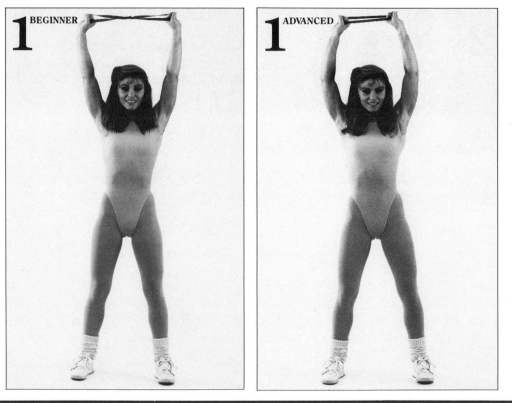

REPETITIONS
Beginner: 8 to 12 for each arm
Advanced: 12 to 16 for each arm

This exercise can also be done in the basic sitting position.

BEGINNER: Basic standing position. Hold the ends of the double band in two fist grips, palms in or out, and raise the arms above the head. The elbows are straight but not locked. Continue with steps 2 and 3.

ADVANCED: Basic standing position. Hold the single band with two fist grips, palms in or out, and raise the arms above the head. The elbows are straight but not locked.

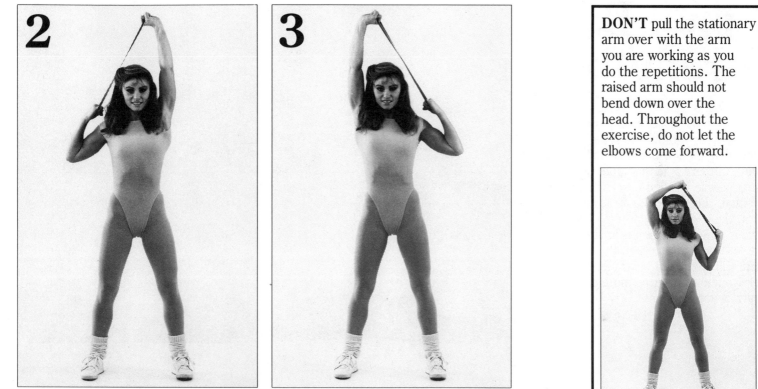

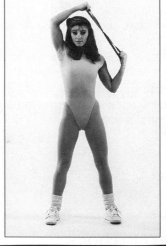

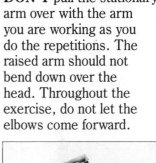

DON'T pull the stationary arm over with the arm you are working as you do the repetitions. The raised arm should not bend down over the head. Throughout the exercise, do not let the elbows come forward.

Keep the left arm raised. Pull the right fist down to shoulder level and slowly raise it back up to the starting position.

Keep the right arm raised. Pull the left fist down to shoulder level and slowly raise it back up to the starting position. Alternate arms as you do the exercise, keeping the repetitions smooth, continuous, and controlled.

Upper Back Strengthener

This is a good, basic exercise to strengthen the upper back, and it can be done with or without the band, depending on how much flexibility and strength there is in the upper body. Most people will find that from a prone position, the closer the arms are to the ears, the harder they are to lift together. If your range of motion is limited, the single band or, if needed, the double band will give you an extra extension to help you hold the arms more comfortably apart as you lift them.

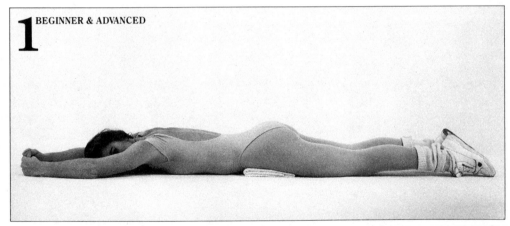

1 BEGINNER & ADVANCED

REPETITIONS
Beginner: 8 to 12
Advanced: 12 to 16

BEGINNER & ADVANCED: In the basic prone position, hold either the double or the single band in two fist grips, depending on individual flexibility. Palms can be in or out, whichever is more comfortable. To take pressure off the lower back, place a folded towel or small pillow under the hips.

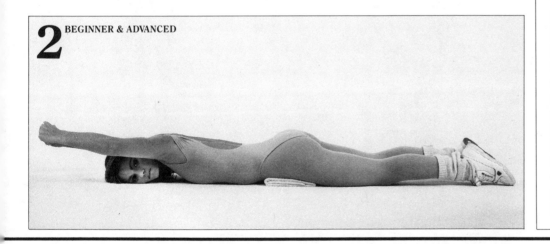

2 BEGINNER & ADVANCED

THE UPPER BACK MUSCLE is located between the shoulder blades—the two "wing" bones in the upper back—and connected right below your neck to about the middle of your back along the spine. Its partner, or opposing muscle, is the chest. It is important to keep the upper back strong to balance it off against the strength of the chest. If the upper back is weak, it gives in to the stronger chest muscles, pulling the upper body forward so it hunches over.

Keep the entire body (including your head) relaxed and on the floor. Lift both arms off the floor as high as you can. Hold for two counts, and release the arms down. Lift and release, keeping the repetitions smooth, continuous, and controlled. Breathe comfortably throughout the exercise: inhale as you release the arms down; exhale as you raise them.

Upright Row

This is the same exercise you would do on a rowing or weight machine to work the upper back with shoulder muscles assisting. Body positions determine the amount of tension in the band: sitting down will give less resistance; standing will give more.

• The whole arm moves throughout this exercise.

• Look away from the rubber band in case it should slip loose or break.

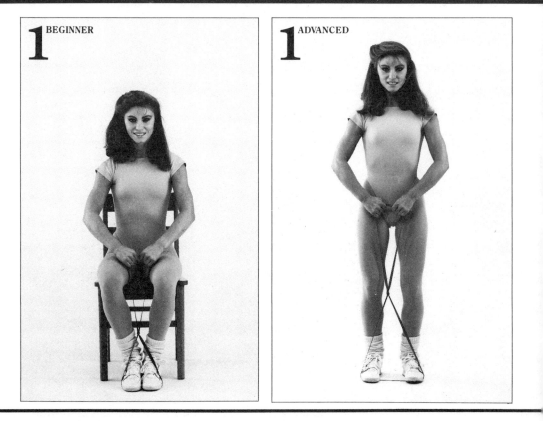

1 BEGINNER

1 ADVANCED

REPETITIONS
Beginner: 8 to 12
Advanced: 12 to 16

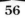

BEGINNER: Basic sitting position. Place the feet through one end of the double band, positioning the band under the arches of the feet, and step down on it. Hold the other end of the band in two fist grips, palms in, elbows bent. Continue with steps 2 and 3.

ADVANCED: Basic standing position. Place the feet through one end of the double band, positioning the band under the arches of the feet, and step down on it. Hold the other end of the band in two fist grips, palms in.

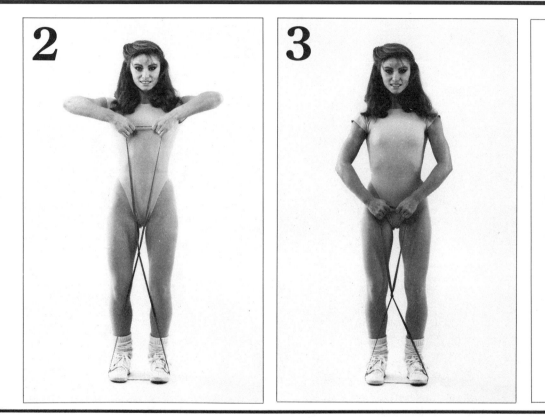

FINE TUNING

Hand and arm positions play an important part in determining which muscles in the upper body are going to get the workout. To feel what happens when you change the angle of the hand, place the left palm on the front of the upper right arm, make a gentle fist with the right hand and bring the forearm up. Now rotate the forearm and feel the way the muscle moves under your palm. Each exercise in The Rubber Band Workout makes use of these subtle changes in position. Upright rows are a good example. With the elbows out to the side, the shoulder and back muscles are worked. However, if the elbows are held close to the side, the area worked shifts to the front of the arm and back muscles.

Pull the band up to chest level. The elbows bend out to the side and both arms move in one smooth motion.

Release the arms down but do not allow slack in the band. Pull up and release down, keeping the repetitions smooth, continuous, and controlled.

Chest Crossover

A small movement in the arms against the resistance of the band creates an effective chest exercise. If it is more comfortable, do this exercise with the band held below chest level.

• Keep the wrists in line with the forearms throughout the exercise.

• Discontinue this exercise if you feel any discomfort in the back.

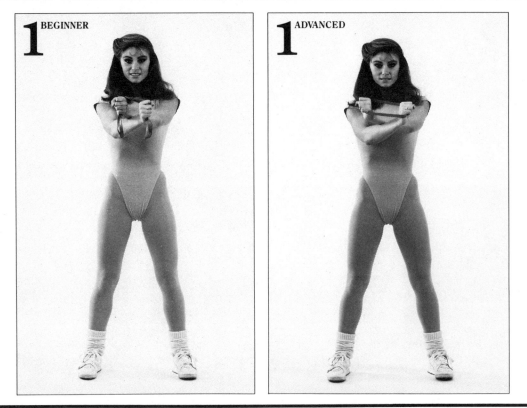

REPETITIONS
Beginner: 8 to 12
Advanced: 12 to 16

This exercise can also be done in the basic sitting position.

BEGINNER: Basic standing position. Hold the double band on each side of the knot in fists, palms in. Cross the forearms, keeping the elbows bent and up at shoulder level. The hands are now back to back, palms out. Continue with steps 2 and 3.

ADVANCED: Basic standing position. Hold the single band out in front of the chest in two fist grips, palms in. Cross the forearms, keeping the elbows bent and up at shoulder level. The hands are now back to back, palms out.

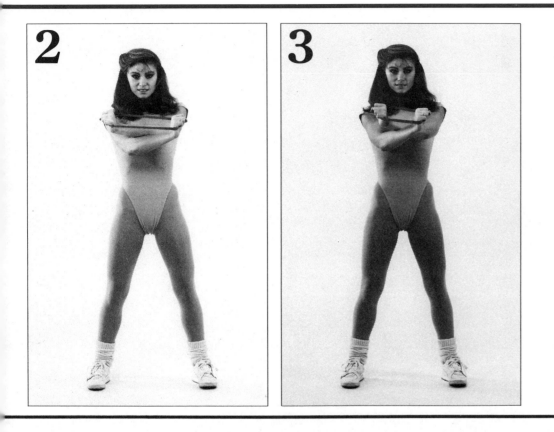

With forearms crossed, slowly press the fists out. Feel the chest muscles work.

Release the fists in, without allowing slack in the band. Press out and release in, keeping the repetitions smooth, continuous and controlled.

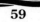

All-Around Chest Conditioner

This is a deceptively simple but highly effective exercise for chest muscles. It is essential, however, that palms face out, arms remain at chest level and wrists are in line with the forearm.

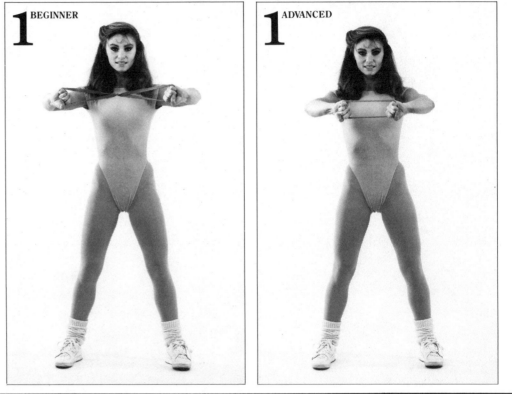

REPETITIONS
Beginner: 8 to 12
Advanced: 12 to 16

This exercise can also be done in the basic sitting position.

BEGINNER: Basic standing position. Hold the ends of the double band in two fist grips, palms out, and arms at chest level. Continue with steps 2 and 3.

ADVANCED: Basic standing position. Hold the single band in two fist grips, palms out, and arms at chest level.

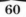

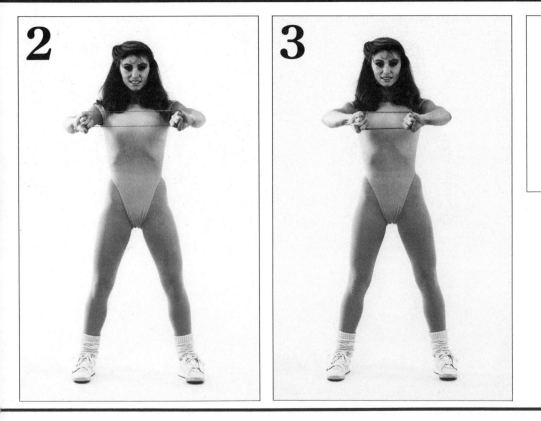

THE CHEST is a push muscle; its partner is the upper back. Put your hand over the breastbone and push your arm out in front. What you feel under your hand is the chest muscle. When you exercise the chest, the assisting muscles will be the back of the arms, or triceps, and the upper back.

Keep the elbows slightly bent. Slowly press the arms out as far as they can comfortably go.

Release the arms in nearly, but not quite, to the starting position and without letting the band go slack. Press out and release in, keeping the band tensed and the repetitions smooth, continuous, and controlled.

Chest Conditioner #2

In this exercise, as well as in the all-around chest conditioner, the chest muscles do most of the work but the shoulder muscles and triceps assist.

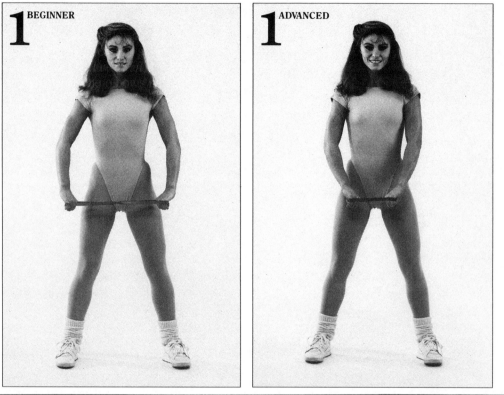

REPETITIONS
Beginner: 8 to 12
Advanced: 12 to 16

This exercise can also be done in the basic sitting position.

BEGINNER: Basic standing position. Hold the double band in two fist grips, palms out, with arms straight down. Keep the elbows slightly bent and the shoulders relaxed down. Continue with steps 2 and 3.

ADVANCED: Basic standing position. Hold the single band in two fist grips, palms out, with arms straight down. Keep the elbows slightly bent and the shoulders relaxed down.

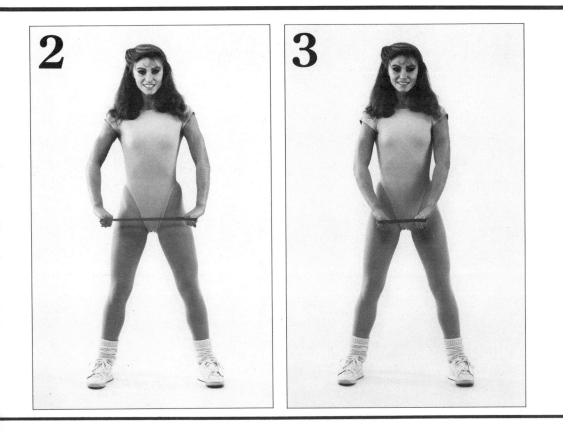

2

3

VARIATION: If you do this exercise in a sitting position, spread the knees apart to allow space for the arms to work. Beginners may use the single band if the double band does not provide enough resistance, but only a little stretch in the band is needed for the exercise to be effective. Do not hunch over; sit comfortably with feet flat on the floor.

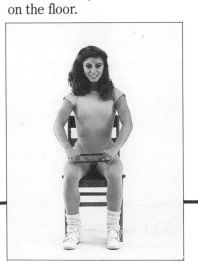

Slowly press the arms out as far as they comfortably go.

Slowly release the arms in nearly, but not quite, to the starting position and without letting the band go slack. Press out and release in, keeping the repetitions smooth, continuous, and controlled.

Shoulder Press-Up

Place a hand on one shoulder and feel the muscles when the arm moves to the side, to the front of the body, toward the back and overhead. Strengthening these muscles can help to improve appearance—strong, well-defined shoulders can make the waist and hips appear smaller, provided we show them off with good posture.

• Be sure the whole arm moves as it presses up.

• Keep the wrist in line with the forearm throughout the exercise.

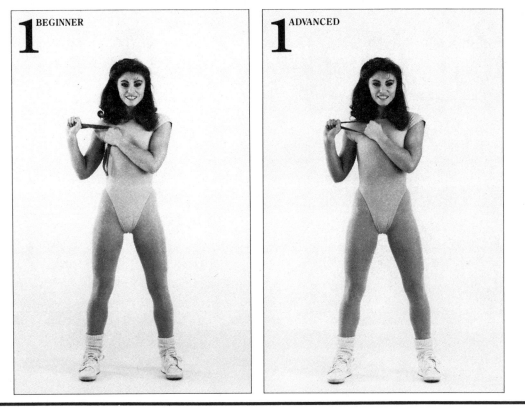

REPETITIONS
Beginner: 8 to 12 for each arm
Advanced: 12 to 16 for each arm

This exercise can also be done in the basic sitting position.

BEGINNER: Basic standing position. Hold the double band below the knot in the left fist, palm in, and place it on the chest at armpit level on the right side. Hold the end of the top loop in a right fist grip, palm forward. Continue with step 2.

ADVANCED: Basic standing position. Hold one end of the single band in a left fist grip, palm in, and place it on the chest at armpit level on the right side. Hold the other end of the band in a right fist grip, palm forward.

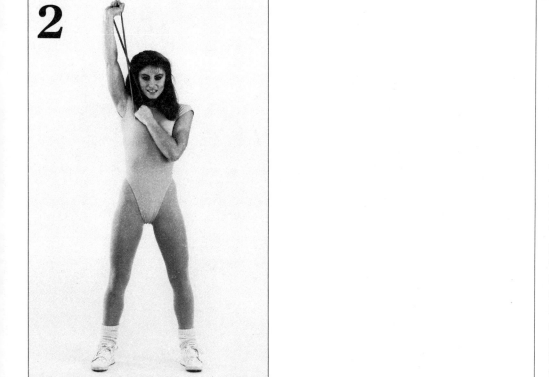

2

Keep the left hand on the chest at armpit level. Press the right arm up toward the ceiling, directly over the right shoulder. Bring the whole arm into the movement and do not lock the elbow. Slowly release the palm down. Press up and release down, keeping the repetitions smooth, continuous, and controlled. Reverse hand positions and repeat the exercise with the left arm.

Shoulder Lat Raise

The "lats" are the muscles that run from the armpits down to the middle of the back, connecting along the spine. In this exercise, shoulder, upper back, and lats work together against the resistance of the band.

• Beginners can adjust the tension in the band by holding it above the knot for more resistance or below the knot for less.

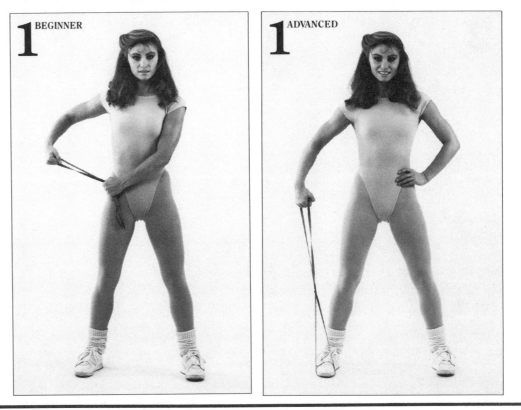

REPETITIONS
Beginner: 8 to 12 for each arm
Advanced: 12 to 16 for each arm

BEGINNER: Basic standing position. Hold the double band at the knot with the left fist, palm in, and place it against the right side of the body. Hold the end of the top loop in a right fist grip, palm down, and elbow out to the side. Continue with steps 2 and 3.

ADVANCED: Basic standing position. Place one end of the double band under the middle of the right foot, at the arch, and step down on it. Hold the other end in a right fist grip, palm down. Bend the elbow slightly.

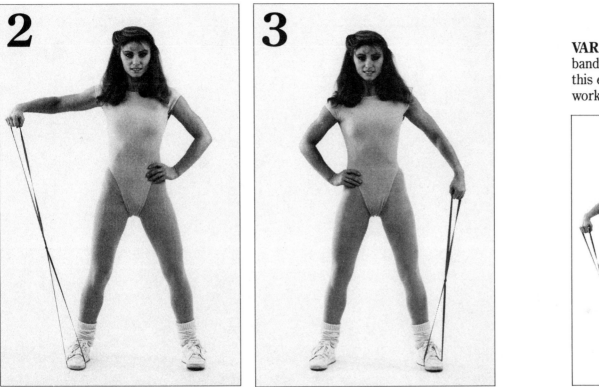

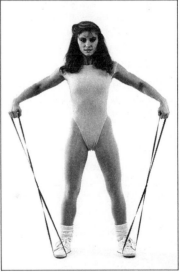

VARIATION: With a double band on each side, you can do this exercise with both arms working simultaneously.

Slowly lift the right arm up to shoulder level. Release the arm partway down, without allowing the band to go slack. Lift up and release, keeping the repetitions smooth, continuous, and controlled.

Reverse positions and repeat the exercise with the left arm.

Shoulder Press-Out

In this exercise, the back muscles assist as both shoulder muscles work together against the resistance of the band. Shoulder press-outs help strengthen the shoulders for better posture.

• Be sure not to overdo this exercise at first. If you feel any discomfort holding the band overhead, relax the arms down and rest them for a few moments before continuing.

• If you feel any discomfort in the shoulder joints, particularly when using the single band, reposition the band as shown in the exercise variation on the facing page. If pain persists, discontinue the exercise.

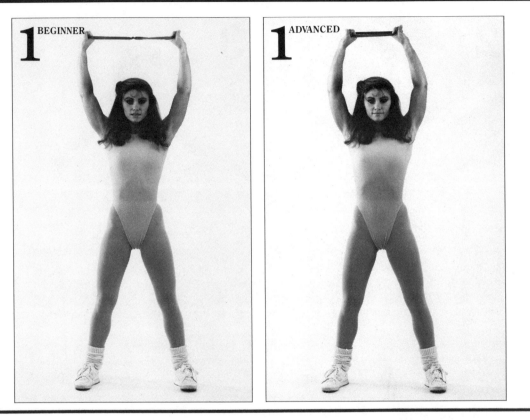

REPETITIONS
Beginner: 8 to 12
Advanced: 12 to 16

This exercise can also be done in the basic sitting positon.

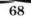

BEGINNER: Basic standing position. Hold the double band overhead in two fist grips, palms out. Keep the shoulders relaxed down, the arms straight but not locked, and the wrists in line with the forearms. Maintain arm position throughout. Continue with steps 2 and 3.

ADVANCED: Basic standing position. Hold the single band overhead in two fist grips, palms out. Keep the shoulders relaxed down, the arms straight but not locked, and the wrists in line with the forearms. Maintain arm position throughout.

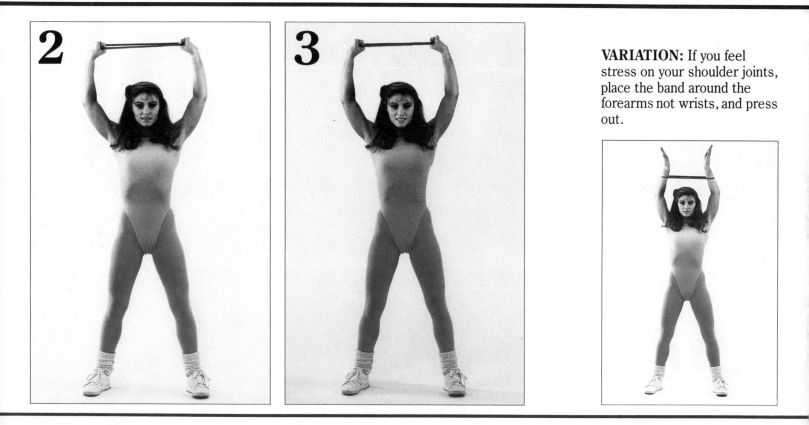

VARIATION: If you feel stress on your shoulder joints, place the band around the forearms not wrists, and press out.

With elbows slightly bent, slowly press the arms out as far as they comfortably go. Exhale as you press out.

Release the arms back nearly, but not quite, to the starting position. Do not allow slack in the band. Press out and release in, keeping the repetitions smooth, continuous, and controlled.

Shoulder Crossover

Think of what it takes to start a lawnmower; that's the kind of motion needed for this exercise. Shoulders and upper back work together against the tension of the band.

• Be sure to move the whole arm as you pull the arm up to shoulder level. Keep the elbow out to the side.

• Keep the back straight and the shoulders from rounding.

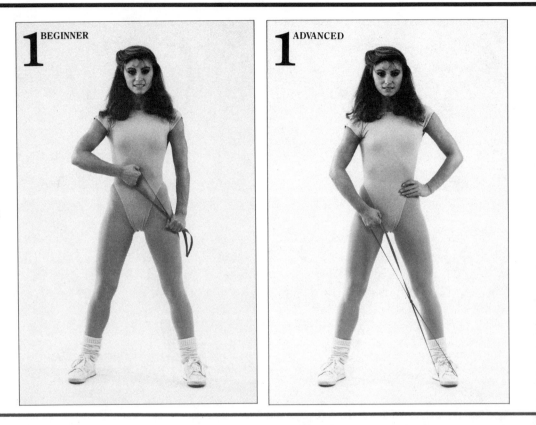

1 BEGINNER

1 ADVANCED

REPETITIONS
Beginner: 8 to 12 for each arm
Advanced: 12 to 16 for each arm

BEGINNER: Basic standing position. Hold the double band below the knot with the left fist, palm in, and place it on the left side at upper thigh level. Hold the end of the top loop of the band in a right fist grip, palm in, and about waist level. Continue with steps 2 and 3.

ADVANCED: Basic standing position. Place one end of the double band under the left foot, at the arch, and step down on it. Hold the other end of the band in a right fist grip, palm in. Bend the elbow up and out to the side, to the point where there is no slack in the band.

2

3

VARIATION: Beginners who feel too much resistance in the standing position can do the exercise seated. Here the point of resistance changes as the band is placed under the foot. For some, this is a more comfortable way to do the exercise than holding the band at the waist.

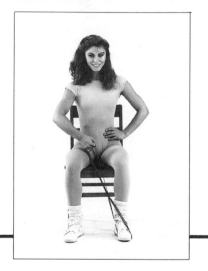

Pull the band across the body to about armpit level on the right side, as if you were starting a lawnmower. Slowly release the band down. Pull across and release down, keeping the repetitions smooth, continuous, and controlled.

Reverse positions and repeat the exercise with the left arm.

Beginner Abdominal Curl, Without the Band

If you have never worked the abdominal muscles in a regular exercise routine, put the band aside for now—the weight of the body will provide more than enough resistance in the exercise given here.

• Exhale as you lift up (the hard part); inhale as you release down (the easy part).

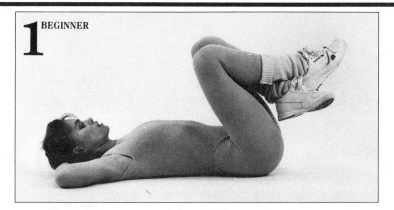

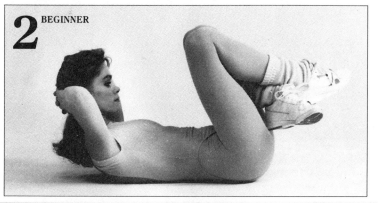

**REPETITIONS
8 to 12**

BEGINNER: Basic floor position, back flat on the floor, hands behind the head. Cross the ankles and draw the knees up toward the chest *(top)*. Slowly raise the upper body toward your knees, trying to lift so that the shoulder blades are off the floor *(bottom)*. Hold for a moment, and slowly lower the upper body to starting position. Lift and lower, keeping the repetitions smooth, continuous, and controlled.

Beginner Reverse Abdominal Curl, Without the Band

If beginner abdominal curls are too difficult, start with reverse abdominal curls, lifting the lower body instead of the upper body.

• Your breathing pattern can help you do this exercise. Exhale as you curl in (the hard part); inhale as you release down (the easy part).

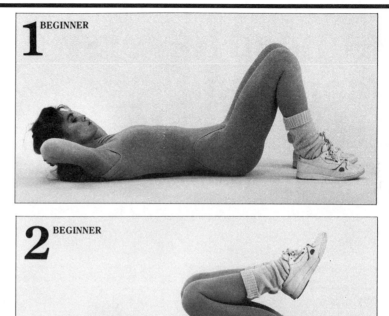

REPETITIONS
8 to 12

BEGINNER: Basic floor position, back flat on the floor and hands behind the head. Bend the knees so the feet are on the floor *(top)*. Slowly curl the knees in toward the chest *(bottom)*. Lower the knees, but no farther than hip level. Do not drop the feet to the floor. Curl in and lower, keeping the repetitions smooth, continuous, and controlled.

Advanced Reverse Abdominal Curl, with the Band

When the beginner curls, without the band, become too easy, move on to the advanced abdominal exercises. The movement of the body is small but with the band this exercise is a big workout for the abdominals.

• If you feel any pain in the back, discontinue the exercise.

• Keep the lower body in the starting position during the exercise.

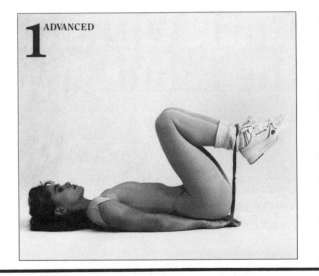

1 ADVANCED

REPETITIONS
Advanced: 8 to 12
Very Advanced: 12 to 16

ADVANCED: Basic floor position, with back flat on the floor. Place one end of the double band around the ankles and bend the knees up to hip level. Hold the other end of the band in two fist grips, palms down, and anchor it under the buttocks. Continue with step 2.

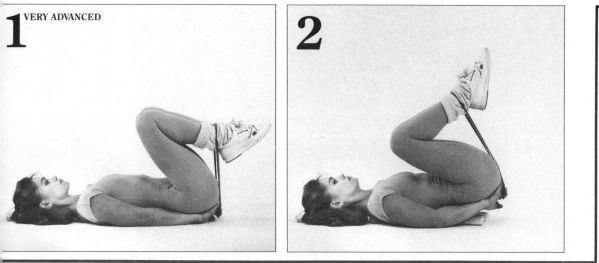

1 VERY ADVANCED

2

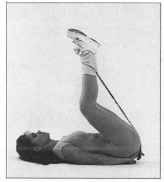

DON'T throw your legs forward and back. Think of curling them in. The knees should not drop past the hips.

VERY ADVANCED: Basic floor position, with back flat on the floor. Place one end of the single band around the ankles and bend the knees up to hip level. Hold the other end of the band in two fist grips, palms down, and anchor it under the buttocks.

Curl the knees in toward the chest and release them back to hip level. Curl in and release, keeping the repetitions smooth, continuous, and controlled.

Abdominal Crossover

As with abdominal curls and sit-ups, beginners will find that the weight of the body is all the resistance needed for the abdominal crossovers. Wait until this exercise becomes too easy before adding the band.

• Exhale as you lift up (the hard part); inhale as you release down (the easy part).

• Concentrate on using the abdominal muscles. Don't let the hands pull up the head and do all the work.

• For added tension, cross the band under the back from the left foot to the right hand or the right foot to the left hand and do your repetitions.

1 BEGINNER

REPETITIONS
Beginner: 8 to 12 on each side
Advanced: 12 to 16 on each side

BEGINNER: Basic floor position, back flat on the floor and hands laced and behind the head. Bend the knees and place the feet on the floor.

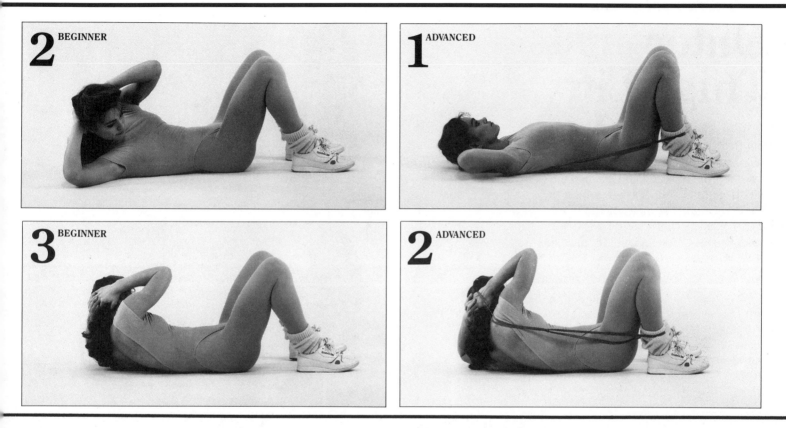

Lift the upper body and cross the left elbow over in the direction of the right knee *(top)*. Lower the body but not quite all the way to the floor. Lift and lower, keeping the repetitions smooth, continuous, and controlled. Repeat the exercise on the other side *(bottom)*.

ADVANCED: Basic floor position, back flat on the floor. Place one end of the double band around the right ankle. Hold the other end in the right fist, and bring the hands up under the head *(top)*. Lift the upper body in the direction of the left knee *(bottom)*. Lower the body, but not quite to the floor. Lift and lower, keeping the repetitions smooth, continuous, and controlled. Repeat the exercise on the other side.

Outer Thigh Lift

Many people think thigh lifts will result in thin thighs—the more repetitions, the thinner the thighs. Thigh lifts firm and condition the muscles and balance out the strength of your legs. If getting rid of fat is the goal, aerobics is the most effective way to burn fat. The Rubber Band Workout helps shape the muscles as fat is lost.

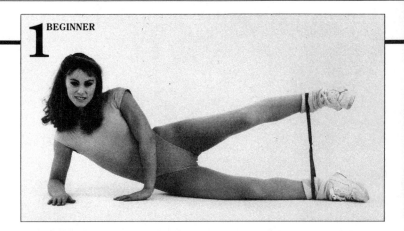

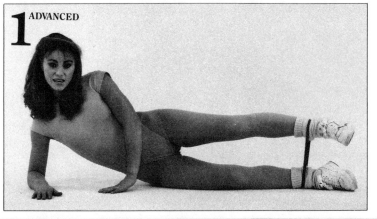

REPETITIONS
Beginner: 8 to 12 for each leg
Advanced: 12 to 16 for each leg

BEGINNER: Basic floor position, lying on one side, top leg slightly raised. Place the double band around both ankles. Continue with steps 2 and 3.

ADVANCED: Basic floor position, lying on one side, top leg slightly raised. Place the single band around both ankles.

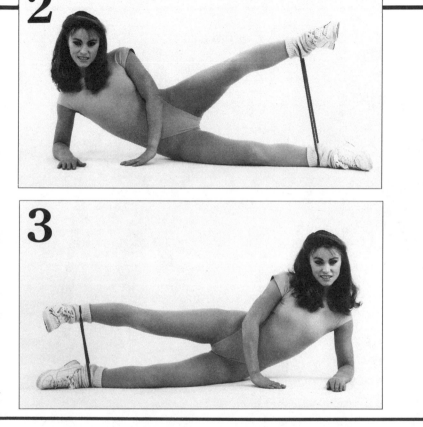

VARIATION: You can do this exercise with the single band placed above the knees, which changes the point of resistance. See if it is more comfortable. This is the preferred position for those with knee problems, because it eliminates pressure on the knee.

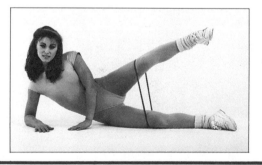

Keeping the foot relaxed (neither flexed nor pointed, but just loose), lift the leg up toward the ceiling as high as possible *(top)*. Slowly lower the leg to the point just before the band goes slack. Lift and lower, keeping the knees and hips facing forward and the repetitions smooth, continuous, and controlled. Change positions and repeat the exercise with the other leg *(bottom)*.

Outer Thigh Lift, Standing

There are several ways to do outer thigh lifts. This exercise is done in the standing position with the band around the ankles or above the knees, whichever is more comfortable.

• Keep the knees and hips facing forward.

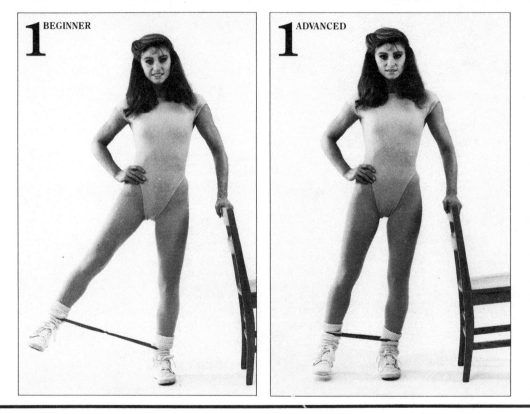

REPETITIONS
Beginner: 8 to 12 for each leg
Advanced: 12 to 16 for each leg

BEGINNER: Basic standing position, one hand holding the back of a chair for support. Place the double band around the ankles. Slightly bend the base leg (nearest the chair) so the knee is not locked. Continue with step 2.

ADVANCED: Basic standing position, one hand holding the back of a chair for support. Place the single band around the ankles. Slightly bend the base leg (nearest the chair) so the knee is not locked.

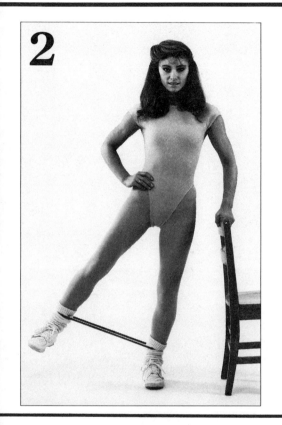

2

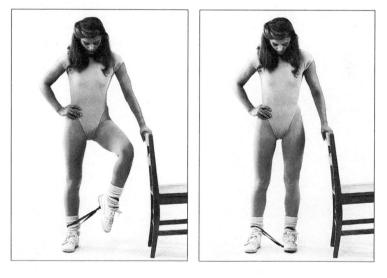

ADDING RESISTANCE

To increase tension in the double band, place it around the ankles; lift the base leg and position the band so that it wraps around the outside of the base foot and under the arch. Step down on the band with the base foot, holding it there throughout the exercise.

Lift the leg out to the side as far as possible; then release the leg, without allowing the band to go slack. Lift the leg to the side and lower, keeping the repetitions smooth, continuous, and controlled. Change sides and do the exercise with the other leg.

Outer Thigh Press-Out

When both thighs are worked together, the muscles in the buttocks, or gluteals, also get a workout.

• This is a very controlled exercise. When you release the knees, be sure they do not flap or snap together. Keep the legs hip level throughout.

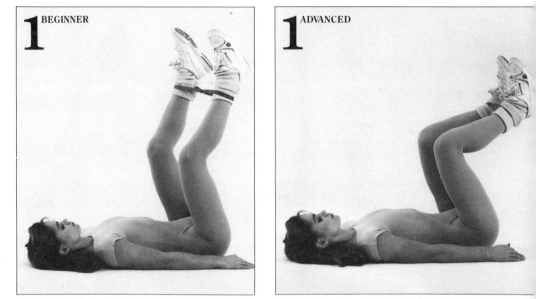

REPETITIONS
Beginner: 8 to 12
Advanced: 12 to 16

BEGINNER: Basic floor position, back flat on the floor and arms at the sides or stretched above the head. Place the double band around the ankles. Bend the knees slightly and draw them up to hip level. Hold this position. Continue with step 2.

ADVANCED: Basic floor position, back flat the floor and arms at the sides or stretched above the head. Place the single band around the ankles. Bend the knees slightly and draw them up to hip level. Hold this position.

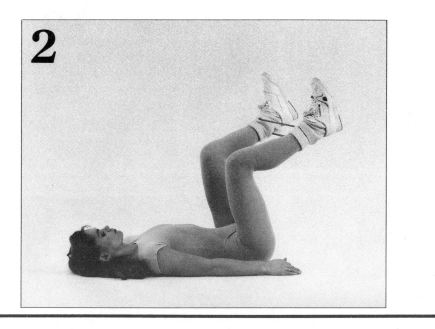

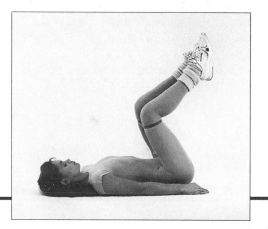

VARIATION: Move the band above the knees to change the point of resistance, especially if pain in the knees occurs, but be sure to wear tights or sweat pants for this position. Do not use the band on bare skin.

Keeping the knees bent, press the legs out. Slowly release them back in, without allowing slack in the band. Press out and release in, keeping the repetitions smooth, continuous, and controlled.

Outer Thigh Press-Out, Seated

This exercise for the outer thighs can be done while sitting at a desk, or traveling, with either bent or straight legs. Most people will prefer to use the single band around the ankles or around the knees, but beginners may want to use the double band at first. Whichever position you choose, don't let the knees flap open or closed.

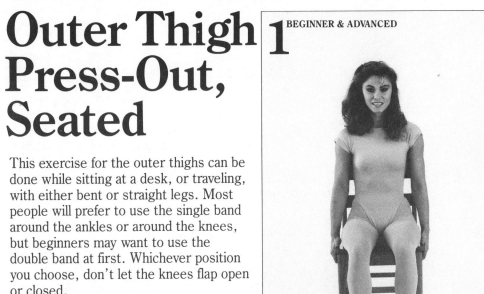

1 BEGINNER & ADVANCED

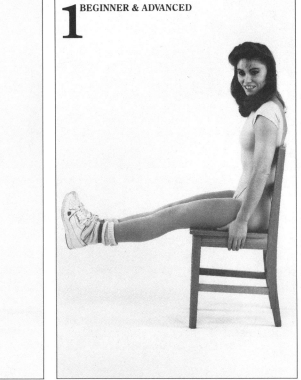

1 BEGINNER & ADVANCED

REPETITIONS
Beginner: 8 to 12
Advanced: 12 to 16

BEGINNER & ADVANCED: Basic sitting position. Place the single or double band around the ankles or above the knees, and hold the edge of the chair for support. Keep the knees bent.

Or keep the legs straight, if that is the position chosen, and the feet flexed.

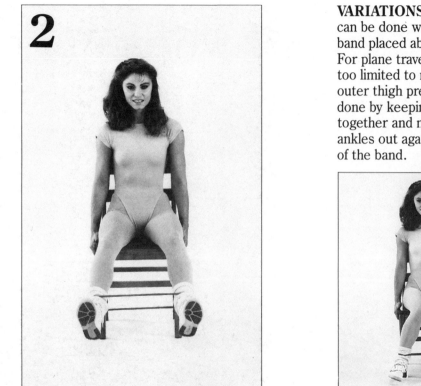

2

VARIATIONS: This exercise can be done with the single band placed above the knees. For plane travel or any space too limited to move the knees, outer thigh press-outs can be done by keeping the knees together and moving the ankles out against the tension of the band.

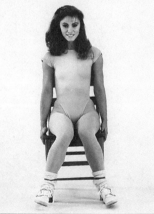

Slowly open the legs to the sides. Release the legs back without allowing slack in the band. Open and release, keeping the repetitions smooth, continuous, and controlled.

Inner Thigh Lift

There are several inner thigh lift exercises, but this one seems to be the favorite. Compared to the outer thigh, the range of movement of the inner thigh is very short. With this and the following inner thigh exercises, the goal is not to see how high you can lift or cross your leg, but rather to concentrate on isolating the inner thigh so that you really feel it working.

• It doesn't matter if the band slides up a little on the leg being worked.

• Do not rotate your hips back. Keep them perpendicular to the floor.

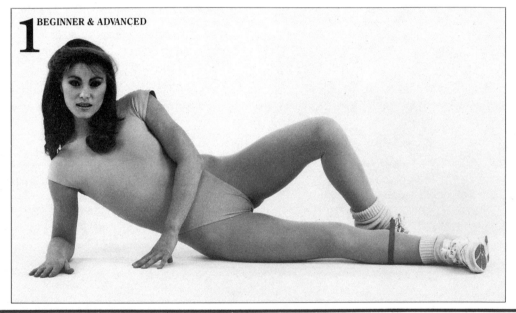

1 BEGINNER & ADVANCED

REPETITIONS
Beginner: 8 to 12 for each leg
Advanced: 12 to 16 for each leg

BEGINNER & ADVANCED: Basic floor position, lying on the right side. Bend the left knee so that the foot is flat on the floor and in back of the right leg. Place one end of the single band around the middle of the left foot and the other end of the band around the right calf. The base leg does not move during the exercise.

VARIATION: The base leg can be placed in front of the leg being exercised. Slowly lift and lower the straight leg in the manner described.

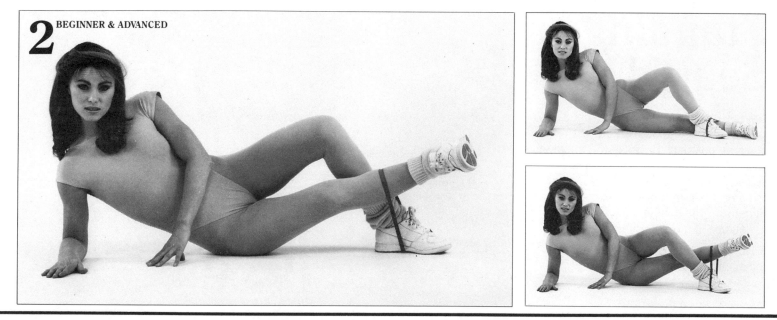

2 BEGINNER & ADVANCED

Slowly lift the right leg up toward the ceiling, keeping the leg straight but not locked, and the knee and hips facing forward. Don't let them roll back. Lower the leg, keeping the band tensed and the foot flexed throughout. Lift and lower, keeping the repetitions smooth, continuous, and controlled. Change sides and repeat the exercise with the left leg.

Inner Thigh Lift, Standing or Seated

Using a chair for balance, the inner thighs can get a good workout in the standing position. Because the range of motion is small, the single band is suggested for beginners, as well as for the advanced, in this exercise. Try it. Substitute the double band if less resistance is more comfortable.

• Do not let the band go slack as you release the foot back.

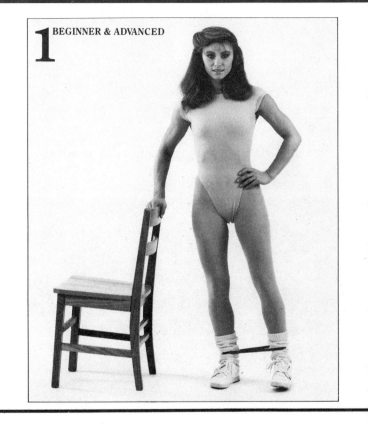

1 BEGINNER & ADVANCED

REPETITIONS
Beginner: 8 to 12 for each leg
Advanced: 12 to 16 for each leg

BEGINNER & ADVANCED: Basic standing position, using the back of a chair for support. Place the single band around the ankles.

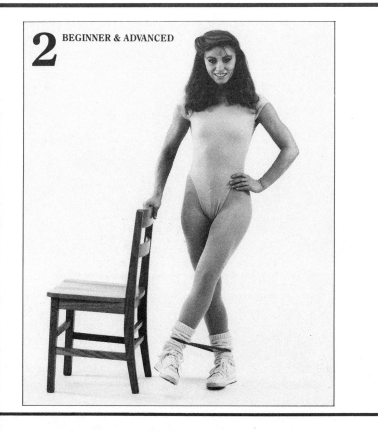

2 BEGINNER & ADVANCED

VARIATION: Do the inner thigh lifts in the basic sitting position, holding the edge of the chair for support. Place the band around the ankles and bring one leg across the front of the body in the manner described. Do the given number of repetitions for your level of strength for each leg.

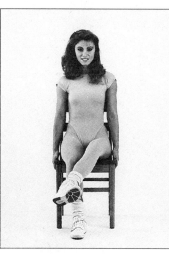

Keeping the left foot flexed and the leg straight, slowly lift the left leg across the body. Slowly release the leg to the starting position. Lift and release, keeping the repetitions smooth, continuous, and controlled. Change sides and repeat the exercise with the right leg.

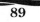

Front of Thigh Extension

This exercise works the front of the thighs, or quadriceps. Nothing moves during the repetitions but the *lower* leg, from the knee joint down. While there are several positions for doing this exercise, lying on the floor is safest for the back, particularly for those who are new to regular exercise or who may have had back injuries.

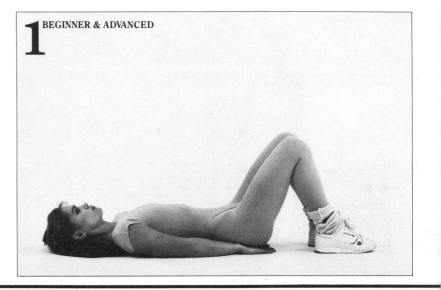

1 BEGINNER & ADVANCED

REPETITIONS
Beginner: 8 to 12 for each leg
Advanced: 12 to 16 for each leg

90

BEGINNER & ADVANCED: Basic floor position, back flat on the floor, knees bent and feet on the floor. Place one end of the double or single band around the right ankle and the other end around the left ankle, adjusting it for more resistance by stepping on it with the left foot (see page 81). For extra support, place the hands under the buttocks.

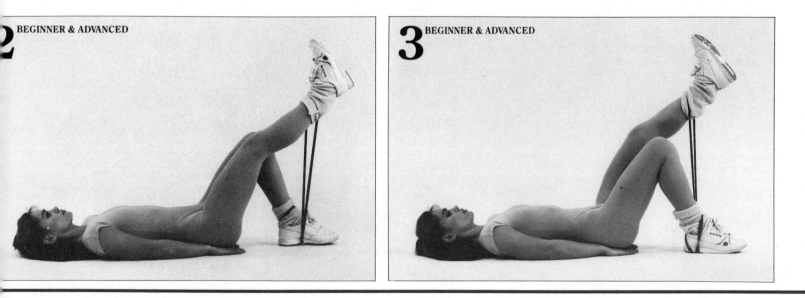

BEGINNER & ADVANCED

Keeping the knees and thighs together, slowly extend the right lower leg as if you were kicking a ball toward the ceiling. Slowly release the leg down, moving just the lower part of the right leg. Extend and release, keeping the repetitions smooth, continuous, and controlled.

Repeat the exercise with the left leg.

Front of Thigh Extension, Standing

Here are two more exercises for the front of the thigh, working one leg at a time and using a chair. Try all the thigh extensions—and vary them in your exercise routine.

• Keep the knee at a 90-degree angle throughout the exercise.

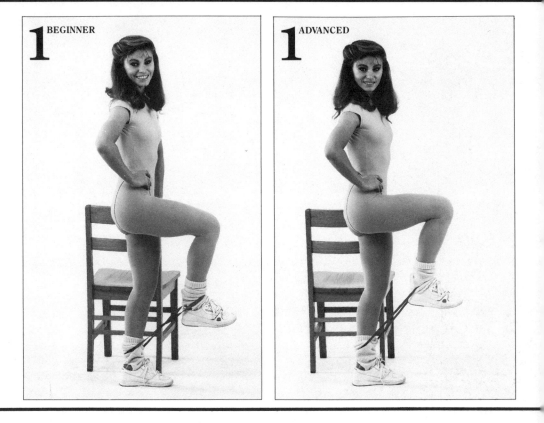

REPETITIONS
Beginner: 8 to 12 for each leg
Advanced: 12 to 16 for each leg

BEGINNER: Basic standing position, holding the back of a chair for balance. Place the double band around the ankles and bend the right knee up to hip level. Hold this position throughout the exercise. Continue with steps 2 and 3.

ADVANCED: Basic standing position, holding the back of a chair for balance. Place the single band around the ankles and bend the right knee up to hip level. Hold this position throughout the exercise.

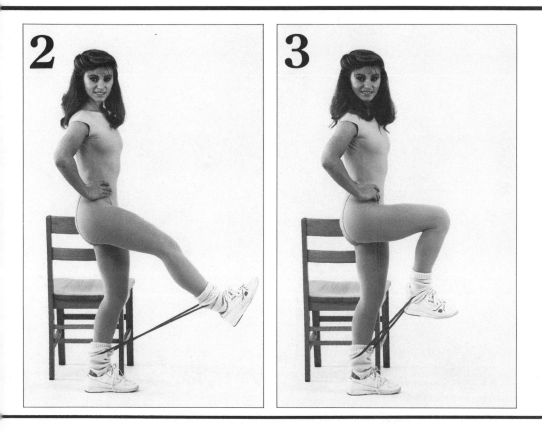

VARIATION: Front of thigh extensions can be done in the basic seated position. Use either the double or the single band, placed around the ankles. Resistance can be increased when using the double band by stepping on one or both sides of it, see page 81. Begin with both feet on the floor and extend the lower leg to knee level.

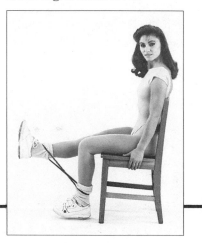

Slowly extend the right leg forward, keeping the knee up and the foot flexed.

Moving only the lower leg, release the right leg to the starting position. Extend and release, keeping the repetitions smooth, continuous, and controlled.

Two-Leg Extension

The fronts of the thighs can also be worked together, with the double band anchored under the buttocks to create a new point of resistance. Keep both knees raised to about waist level as you move only the lower legs.

• Keep the feet flexed to help secure the band.

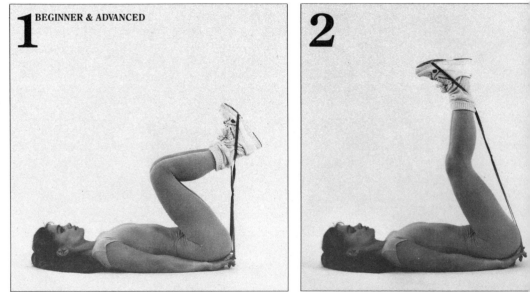

1 BEGINNER & ADVANCED

2

REPETITIONS
Beginner: 8 to 12
Advanced: 12 to 16

BEGINNER & ADVANCED: Basic floor position, back flat on the floor. Bend the knees up to hip level and place one end of the double band around the bottom of the feet, at the arch. Hold the other end of the band in two fist grips, palms down, and place them under the buttocks.

Keeping the knees up to about waist level and the feet flexed, extend the lower legs as far as they will go.

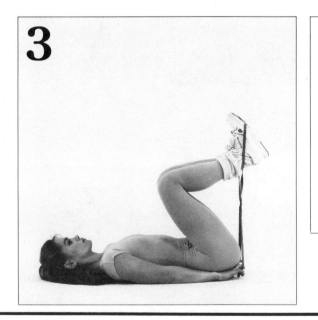

3

THE QUADRICEPS, located on the front of the thigh, includes four major muscles that extend from the hip down to the kneecap. Place your hand on your thigh and extend your leg out. What you feel working underneath your hand is the quadriceps. When you concentrate on moving nothing but the lower leg, it isolates the front of the thigh during the exercise.

Slowly release the legs to the starting position, without allowing any slack in the band. Extend and release, keeping the repetitions smooth, continuous, and controlled.

Back of Thigh Curl, Prone Position

A lift is quite a different movement from a curl. For the latter, a certain part of the body (arm, leg, upper or lower torso) is curled in toward an imaginary point at the center of the body. A lift is just that, lifting a part of the body against its own weight—or the resistance of the band.

• Think of *curling* the lower leg in toward the center of the body when you do this exercise. Isolate and think about the back of the thigh as it moves.

• Keep the foot flexed as you lift it.

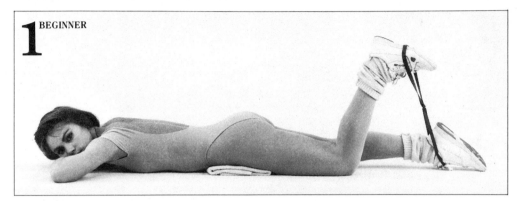

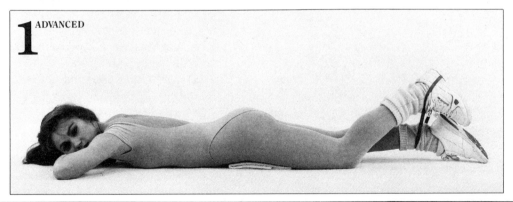

REPETITIONS
Beginner: 8 to 12 for each leg
Advanced: 12 to 16 for each leg

BEGINNER: Basic prone position (*top*). Place one end of the double band around the right ankle and the other end around the arch of the left foot. Continue with steps 2 and 3.

ADVANCED: Basic prone position (*bottom*). Place one end of the single band around the right ankle and the other end around the arch of the left foot.

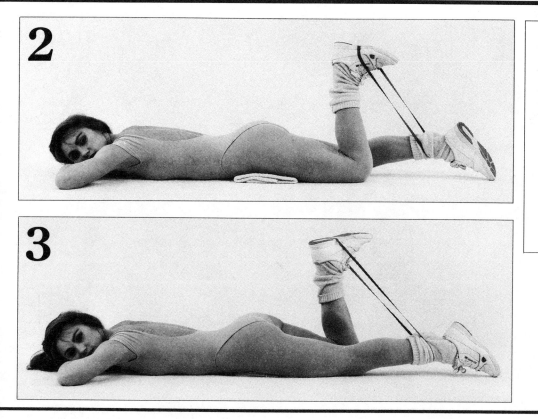

THE HAMSTRINGS on the back of the thigh run from the back of the knee up to the buttocks. These muscles push the body forward when taking a step. As the partner to the very strong muscles on the front of the thigh, the back of the thigh tends to get very tight. It needs conditioning, but it also needs to be stretched. Do the strengthening exercises for the back of the thigh, but also do the stretches beginning on page 116.

Flex the left foot and curl it in toward the buttocks *(top)*. Slowly release the foot down, without allowing slack in the band. Curl in and release down, keeping the repetitions smooth, continuous, and controlled. Reverse band positions and do the exercise with the right leg *(bottom)*.

Back of Thigh Curl, Standing and Seated

As with other exercises in this book, varying the body positions creates options and makes it possible to do the exercises in many situations throughout the day. Here are two variations for working the back of the thigh.

• Remember to keep the foot flexed as the leg moves against the resistance of the band. Keep the knees together.

• Only the lower leg moves during the exercises.

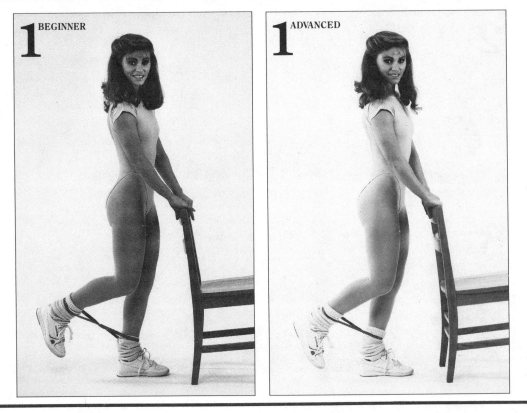

1 BEGINNER

1 ADVANCED

REPETITIONS
Beginner: 8 to 12 for each leg
Advanced: 12 to 16 for each leg

BEGINNER: Basic standing position. Hold the back of a chair for support. Place the double band around the ankles and extend the right leg out in back to create tension in the band. Flex the foot. Continue with step 2.

ADVANCED: Basic standing position. Hold the back of a chair for support. Place the single band around the ankles and extend the right leg out in back to create tension in the band. Flex the foot.

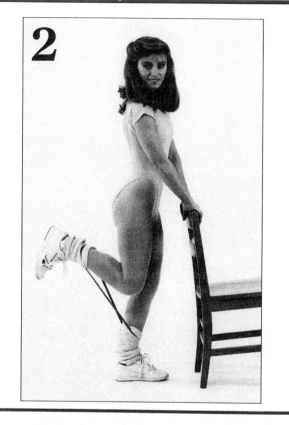

VARIATION: To work the back of the thighs from the basic seated position, place the single band around the ankles and extend the legs out straight. This is the starting position. Keep the knees together and release the left leg down. Raise it up and curl it down—keeping the repetitions smooth, continuous, and controlled. Repeat the exercise with the right leg.

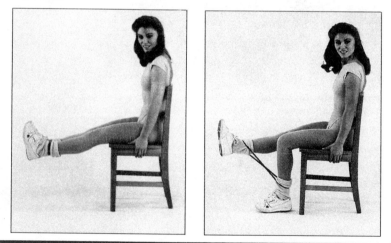

Keeping the foot flexed and the knees together, curl the right leg toward the buttocks. Release the leg back down, but do not let the band go slack. Curl in and release down, keeping the repetitions smooth, continuous, and controlled. Repeat the exercise with the left leg.

Back of Thigh Lift

The back of the thighs will benefit from a simple lift—raising the bent leg slightly off the floor. In this exercise, both the buttocks muscles and the back of the thighs get a workout.

• Only a small lift of the leg is necessary for the back of the thigh to get a workout.

• Keep the raised foot flexed throughout the exercise.

• If lower back pain occurs, discontinue the exercise.

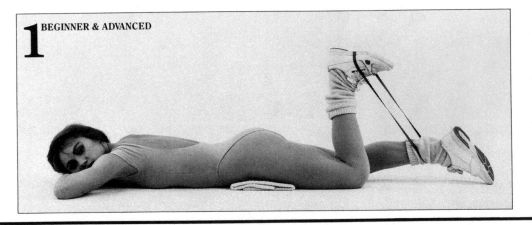

1 BEGINNER & ADVANCED

REPETITIONS
Beginner: 8 to 12 for each leg
Advanced: 12 to 16 for each leg

BEGINNER & ADVANCED: Basic prone position. Place one end of the single band around the right ankle and the other end around the middle of the left foot, at the arch. Bend the left leg up to form a 90-degree angle at the knee. Keep the foot flexed. The leg does not move from this position during the exercise.

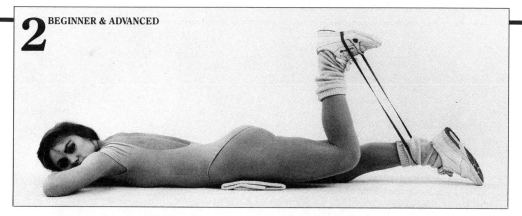

2 BEGINNER & ADVANCED

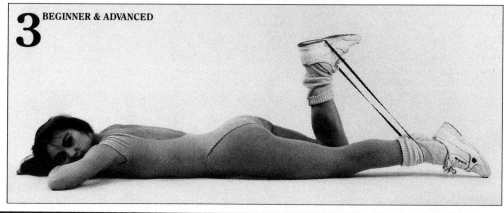

3 BEGINNER & ADVANCED

Squeezing the buttocks together, push the hips down and lift the left leg an inch or so off the floor. Hold for a moment. Feel it in the buttocks and back of thigh. Release the leg down to the floor, but keep the knee bent. Lift the leg and release it down, keeping the repetitions smooth, continuous, and controlled (*top*). Reverse band positions and repeat the exercise with the right leg (*bottom*).

Straight-Leg Lift

Keeping the leg straight as it's lifted in back is another way to work the back of the thighs and the buttocks together. Try to keep the buttocks squeezed together during this exercise.

• Since the range of motion is short, the resistance of the single band is fine for most beginners.

• To eliminate pressure on the lower back, place a towel or small pillow under the hips.

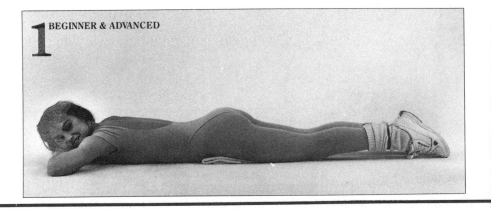

1 BEGINNER & ADVANCED

REPETITIONS
Beginner: 8 to 12 for each leg
Advanced: 12 to 16 for each leg

BEGINNER & ADVANCED: Basic prone position. Place the single band around the ankles (or above the knees to change the point of resistance).

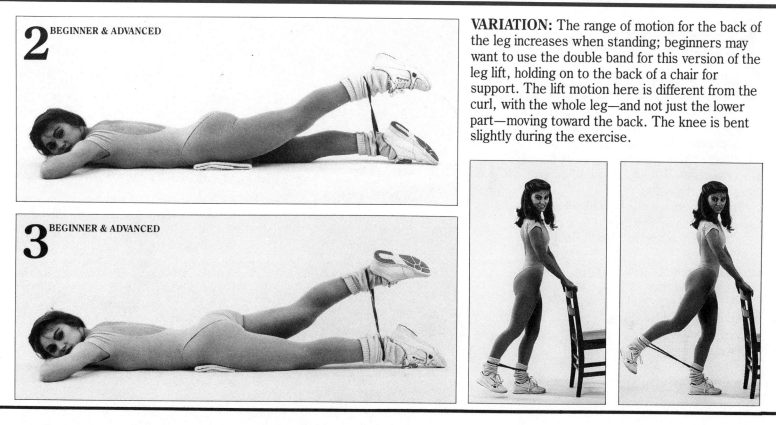

2 BEGINNER & ADVANCED

3 BEGINNER & ADVANCED

VARIATION: The range of motion for the back of the leg increases when standing; beginners may want to use the double band for this version of the leg lift, holding on to the back of a chair for support. The lift motion here is different from the curl, with the whole leg—and not just the lower part—moving toward the back. The knee is bent slightly during the exercise.

With both hips on the floor and the legs straight, slowly lift the left leg. It's a small lift off the floor, but feel it in the back of the thighs and buttocks *(top)*. Slowly lower the leg, without letting the band go slack. Lift and lower, keeping the repetitions smooth, continuous, and controlled. Repeat the exercise with the right leg *(bottom)*.

Hip Flexor Strengthener

The hip flexor is the muscle that connects the front of the hip joint with the thigh. If the abdominals are weak and the lower back is tight, usually the hip flexors are tight, too.

To test whether the hip flexors are tight, lie down on the floor and draw the left knee up toward the chest. Hold it there and extend your right leg, trying to press the back of the right knee to the floor. If it stays raised more than two inches, you should add the hip flexor stretch (page 120) to your regular routine to increase flexibility in this area, as flexibility helps prevent injuries.

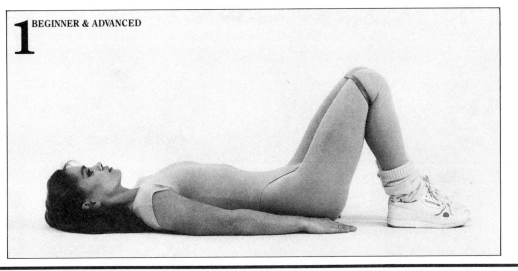

1 BEGINNER & ADVANCED

REPETITIONS
For all: 8 to 12 for each leg

BEGINNER & ADVANCED: Basic supine position, with knees bent, feet together on the floor and arms at the side. Place the single band above both knees.

VARIATION: To do this exercise standing up, use the back of a chair for support and place the single band around the ankles. Draw the knee up to hip level, keeping the foot flexed as the leg is raised.

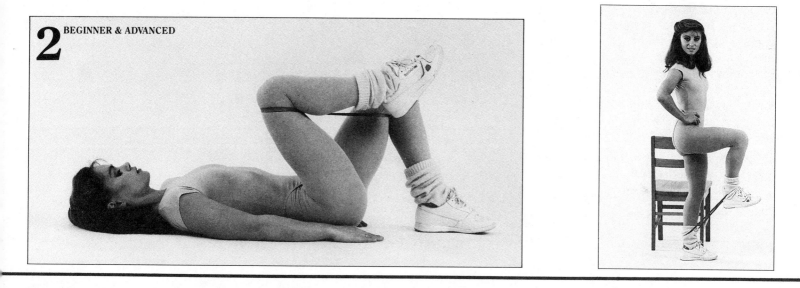

2 BEGINNER & ADVANCED

Slowly bring the right knee in toward your chest. Release it back down. Bring the knee in and release down, keeping the repetitions smooth, continuous, and controlled. Repeat the exercise with the left leg.

Shin Strengthener

"Shin splints" occur when the calves are tight and put stress on the shin bone, the shin muscle, and the tendons connecting the muscle to the bone. This exercise can help prevent this common discomfort—by strengthening and stretching the muscles at the front of the lower legs. There are three variations to choose from, with the single band used throughout.

• Be sure to place the band high on the shoe so it will not slip off.

• Only the top foot moves as you do the repetitions.

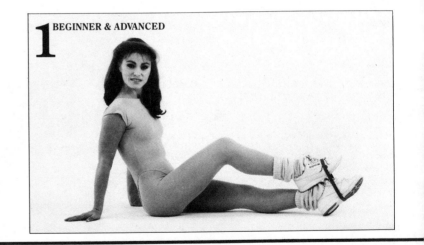

1 BEGINNER & ADVANCED

REPETITIONS
For all: 8 to 12 for each leg

This exercise can also be done in the basic sitting position.

BEGINNER & ADVANCED: Sit on the floor with legs extended, hands behind you for support. Place the single band around the middle of the feet, at the arches. Move the right leg up so the right heel is resting on the side of the left shin, near the ankle. Hold it there.

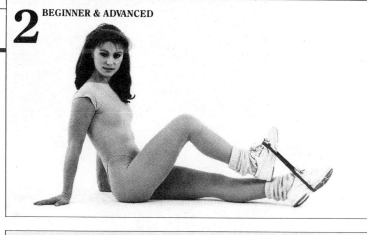

2 BEGINNER & ADVANCED

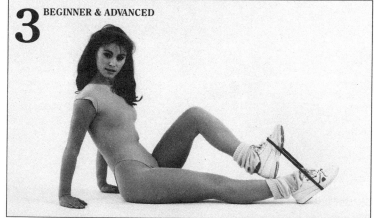

3 BEGINNER & ADVANCED

VARIATION: The floor position is the same as in the main exercise, but the feet are worked together. Place the single band around the middle of both feet, keeping the feet flexed (toes pointed up) and the heels together on the floor *(left)*. Open the feet *(right)* and close. Do the same number of repetitions given for the main exercise.

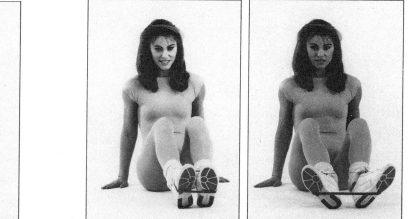

Curl the right foot in toward the body, keeping the heel in position on the left shin *(top)*. Slowly release the foot down. Curl in and release down, keeping the repetitions smooth, continuous, and controlled. Reverse the positions of the feet and do the exercise with the left foot *(bottom)*.

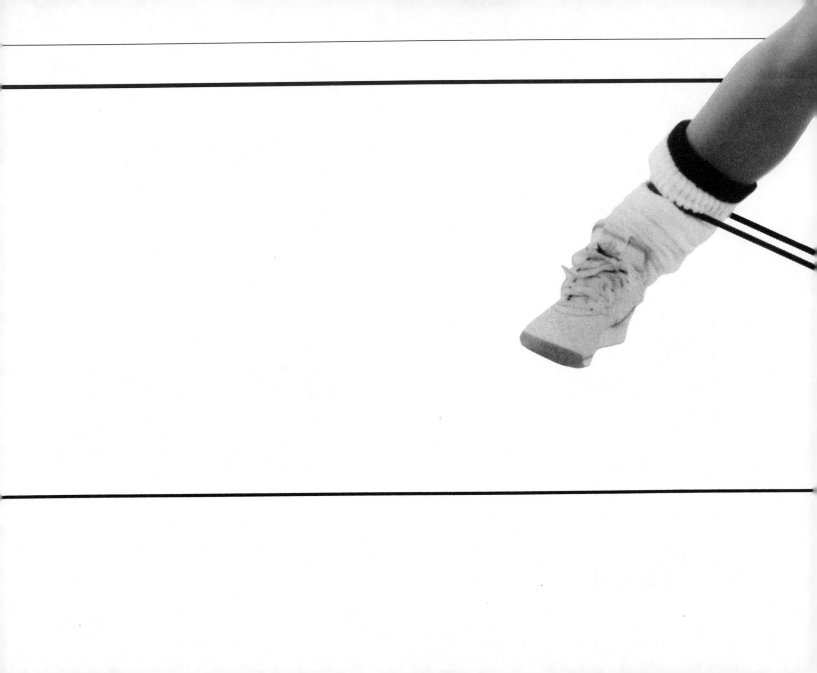

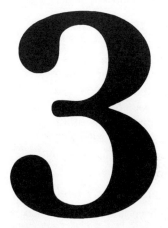

3

THE RUBBER BAND WORKOUTS:

FIVE CUSTOMIZED PROGRAMS FOR THE BEGINNER TO THE VERY ADVANCED

THE RUBBER BAND WORKOUTS

START WITH YOUR DOCTOR'S APPROVAL

It's important to get a physical checkup and your doctor's approval before starting a new fitness program. This goes for The Rubber Band Workout and for any other form of exercise, especially for:

• Those who have *never routinely exercised* before;

• Those who are *very overweight*;

• Those who have had *back problems;*

• Those who may have a *heart condition* (get a checkup to be sure your heart is healthy, especially if you include aerobics in your fitness program, as aerobics works the heart);

• Those who may have *high blood pressure* (when you work with any type of resistance, your blood pressure will go up, so if you have high blood pressure you should not begin this resistance program until your blood pressure is confirmed normal by a doctor).

The workouts in this section of the book are designed for all levels of fitness and tailored to a variety of lifestyles. Choose the program that best fits your needs and the time you have to give to it. Change or alter the program when it becomes necessary. That way, you will have a workout for today, next week, and all through the year—no matter how your schedule may vary or your needs change.

The Get-in-Shape and Stay-in-Shape workouts are complete programs as they combine aerobics (with a warm-up period before and a cool-down period after) and a stretch sequence with the resistance exercises. The Get-in-Shape Workout suggests one resistance exercise per muscle group, whereas the Stay-in-Shape Workout increases to two exercises per group. These two complete programs, when done three to five days a week, are highly recommended for achieving long-term fitness goals.

THE WORKOUTS	TIME REQUIRED
The Beginner or Get-in-Shape Workout	½ to 1 hour, 3 days per week, 2 to 4 weeks or longer (depending on the progress of the individual)
The Stay-in-Shape Workout	½ to 1 hour, 3 to 4 days per week, ongoing
The Ten-Minute Workout	10 to 15 minutes, no more than 2 to 3 times per week
The Chair Workout	10 to 15 minutes, no more than 2 to 3 times per week
The Power Workout	½ to 1 hour, 3 to 5 days per week, ongoing

But, if you really *don't* have the time, consider the following alternatives.

The Ten-Minute Workout and The Chair Workout eliminate aerobics. They are geared either for those with only ten minutes, or those whose optimum time for exercise is when they are sitting (i.e., traveling or working at a desk). The Chair Program is ideal for those with certain physical limitations, provided it has their doctor's approval.

The Power Workout is presented as a suggestion for those who are very advanced and want to increase the resistance of the band.

Whichever workout you choose, do the complete resistance program two or three times a week, every *other* day— and no more. However, if you want to work out more often, you can exercise certain muscle groups on one day and other muscle groups the next. Just be sure your muscles get a day of recuperation to rebuild between your workouts.

In customizing your own Rubber Band Workout, you can pick and choose the exercises you like best within each muscle group, or you can follow exactly the suggestions given with each program.

I recommend that you start with the Get-in-Shape Program. When it becomes too easy for you, either add more repetitions or more resistance to the exercises you are doing, or go on the Stay-in-Shape Workout, continuing the beginner program, but adding one or two more exercises per muscle group to the resistance part of the program. Use the double band at first, but when you know you are ready for more of a challenge, move to the single band.

To stay in shape, you must commit yourself to a minimum of three days of exercise a week—it cannot be done with less. Once you've established a regular fitness routine, the best goal is to keep to your program.

Those who are ready for it, who know they are strong because they have been doing resistance for some time and have seen body changes in strength and weight and shape, can begin the Power Workout.

THE ROLE OF AEROBICS AND COOL DOWN

What resistance does to strengthen the muscles, aerobic exercise does to burn off fat. This is a very important analogy and a persuasive argument in favor of the complete programs. Aerobic exercise burns calories during exercise—and even afterward as the body cools down.

Aerobic exercise demands an uninterrupted output from the muscles to utilize oxygen for a minimum of fifteen to twenty minutes (which also increases the body's ability to take in oxygen and improves the cardiovascular system's ability to supply the oxygen and nutrients to the body). Studies prove

THE RUBBER BAND WORKOUTS

that after an initial twenty minutes of aerobics, the body, like a warmed-up engine, operates more smoothly and burns fat more effectively. So if you can push yourself past the twenty minute mark, keep going up to thirty minutes.

Aerobics exercise is endurance exercise, but many people think of aerobics as punishment—doing fifty jumping jacks, or simply jumping up and down until you are breathless, sweaty, and sore. This may be realistic for a marine in bootcamp, but the rest of us can get the benefits of aerobics from more comfortable activities—a brisk walk, using a stationary bike, dancing to music in your living room—as long as you are uninterrupted for fifteen to twenty minutes. It is better to do aerobics at an easy pace for twenty minutes than to do ten minutes at an uncomfortable one. Fat seems to burn more effectively with a longer duration at lower intensity than with a shorter duration at a higher

intensity. If you are unable to talk or carry on a conversation while you are doing aerobics, you are working too hard—slow down.

After you have completed your warm-up and stretches, you are ready for aerobic exercise. As with the warm-up, the increase in heart rate and body movement should be gradual. Begin slowly and work up to a vigorous pace. You do not have to run a marathon or jog ten miles to fulfill the requirement. Remember, fitness is not punishment—it's an award you wear throughout life.

After fifteen to twenty minutes of vigorous aerobics, don't just stop. You need a three- to five-minute cool-down period. It is important to gradually slow your heart rate with less vigorous movements, just as you gradually increased it. Continue your exercise, but ease up until you feel your heart rate return to normal.

FINDING TIME FOR FITNESS

You have to want fitness. Nobody else can achieve it for you. You've got to know your own body, and what it needs. You have to decide how many hours a week you can contribute to your body—to doing the program.

When I design a fitness program for a client, we sit down together and look over his or her appointment book. We look to see where there is some leeway, where we can find a slot for exercise as part of the regular routine.

Ideally, we want to find the time when the body will perform at its best. In the morning? The afternoon? The evening? Think about it. Some people can go to work in the morning and give it all they've got—they are ready to go and the creative juices are flowing. After lunch, they reach a low point, and perhaps pick up again in the evening. Others do not hit their full stride until later in the day, and they can keep right on going through the evening.

Try to determine when you are at your physical peak, and if you have any choice, try to set aside your time for fitness to coincide with it. Is it at lunchtime, and can you squeeze exercise in during a lunch hour? Is it in the morning? If so, can you get up an hour early and do the program? If an hour is too much, then half an hour. Even ten minutes is better than nothing. Block off time for exercise on your calendar, and then stick to it.

TAMILEE'S TIPS FOR HEALTHY EATING HABITS

1. Adjust your appetite to what your body needs. If you are overweight, you have probably conditioned your body to expect more food than it needs. Cut down your extra intake gradually, by putting one less spoonful of food per serving onto your plate until what you eat is slightly less than what you put out as energy burned.

2. Eat on a schedule. Your body likes to know when it is going to be fed. Fix your optimum meal schedule to get your quota of nourishment for the day. Gradually stretch out the time between snacks and when you have pushed them into your meal schedule, eat what your body needs first, wait ten minutes, and then ask yourself if you really want that snack food. If you can live without it, save it for your "treat day."

3. Give yourself a treat day. If you stick to a well-balanced diet all week, you deserve to indulge yourself with a little treat—a chocolate brownie, a slice of cheesecake, whatever you desire in a reasonable portion—on Saturday or Sunday. Savor it!

4. Don't bring junk food into the house, and don't use the excuse that you are buying it for others in the house "who don't need to watch what they eat." They don't need junk food either! Keep tasty, cut-up raw vegetables or your own trail mix—sunflower seeds, raisins, walnuts, almonds, etc.—on hand for snack food.

5. If you are overweight, make one or two pounds a week, not five or ten, your weight-loss goal. Trying to get rid of your extra pounds too quickly will benefit neither your body nor its appearance.

6. Say no to food or coffee when you really don't need it. Most of us are conditioned to accept food when we arrive at someone else's home or office. Next time, before you take it, *really think* about whether you want it or not.

7. Cut out your food obsessions one at a time. Some foods are too painful to give up forever, or even all at once. Phase them out of your eating patterns one at a time, and you'll transform them from obsessions to treats—once in a while.

8. Don't compare your eating habits with those of others. Each body has its own individual needs, its own rate of metabolism, its own tendency to store or burn fat. Recognize how your own body responds to foods, and feed it what will suit you best.

9. Activate your lifestyle and stay out of the kitchen. Plan your meals once a week, and then forget about what you are going to eat. Get involved with the rest of the world and get your mind off food!

10. Reward your body with fitness. Put food into its proper place as the eating part of an overall fitness program. Your reward will be a body that makes you feel good inside because it looks good outside.

THE RUBBER BAND WORKOUTS

WARM-UP

It is best to prepare your body for any major workout. Through a sequence of easy body movements, the body can be readied for any level of exercise it is called upon to do. Simple basic movements bring about an increase in the heart rate and speed the flow of blood through the body. The result is a rise in body temperature, which lubricates the joints and increases muscle elasticity. Warmed muscles can be stretched further, have a wider range of motion and are less likely to tear when worked. Lubricated joints move more easily and take strain off any surrounding tissues.

A brisk walk, light dancing, or just moving energetically around a room will warm the body enough to increase the comfort and effectiveness of the workout. It also decreases the susceptibility to injury.

I include an example of a warm-up sequence. Improvise and adapt it to your own style, but be sure to keep all movements smooth and controlled.

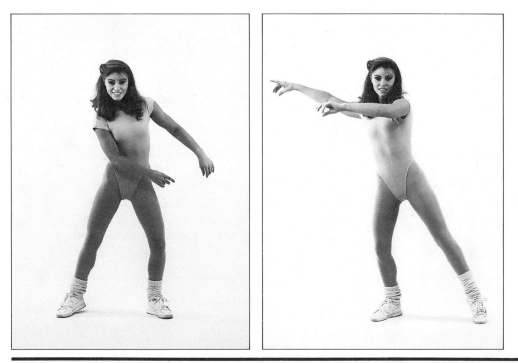

Start with the feet apart and arms to the sides.

Swing the arms gently from side to side . . .

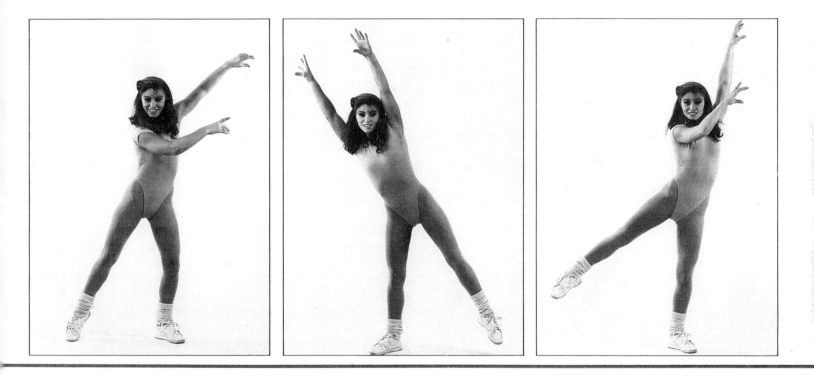

...*gradually reaching higher with each swing.*

Make the motions larger as you swing the arms across the body and higher into the air.

Lift your feet off the floor as you reach to the ceiling. Continue the movements for about five minutes to warm up the body.

THE RUBBER BAND WORKOUTS

STRETCHES

Stretching is a very important part of The Rubber Band Workout. The resistance exercises strengthen the muscles; the stretching exercises keep them flexible, especially after they have been worked so intensely against the resistance of the band. The stretches also keep muscles from tightening up. And, because stretching the limbs gives them a greater range of motion, it also helps prevent injuries—especially when we exercise. The stretching sequence (concentrating on all the muscles being worked) should be done before *and* after The Rubber Band Workout. However, if time is limited, you can warm up the body for three to five minutes or so to get the blood moving throughout the body, skip the stretches, and go right to the resistance exercises. Whether or not you include the stretch sequence before the workout, *always* do it immediately after your resistance exercises.

Even if you miss your regular exercises, make it a point to do the stretches on a daily basis. It's the very least you can do for your body. Remember that as we grow older it is natural for our bodies to shrink and our muscles to tighten up. Stretching helps combat this process. Start your day with stretches—you'll feel relaxed and rested, regardless of how much sleep you've had the night before. Take a break during the day to stretch, particularly those parts of the body you've been holding in the same position for any length of time.

In many exercise programs, stretching is done standing up and bending over from the waist. This is called "forward flexion," but I do not believe this is the safest position for stretching or exercising. This position has a negative effect on the spine and is uncomfortable for most of us. The safest, most comfortable stretching exercises are those that eliminate the pull of gravity and pressure on the back—which is why there are so many floor exercises in this book. Instead of doing the forward flexion stretches, standing up and bending down, you can stretch more comfortably on your back.

Don't bounce when you stretch. Bouncing is called "ballistic stretching"—it helps you stretch to the farthest point. But bouncing teases the muscle, pulling on it, and if that muscle is not warmed up, the muscle tissue may tear. This results in a good deal of pain and a long healing process. Stretches should be slow and easy, and if you would like to do them to music, choose music that relaxes—classical or jazz, for example.

Stretch the muscle to the point of tightness, not to pain; hold and breathe for a count of eight or ten; release; and repeat. That's all there is to it.

THE BASIC TEN-STRETCH SEQUENCE

This stretching sequence includes one exercise for each of the muscle groups involved in The Rubber Band Workout.

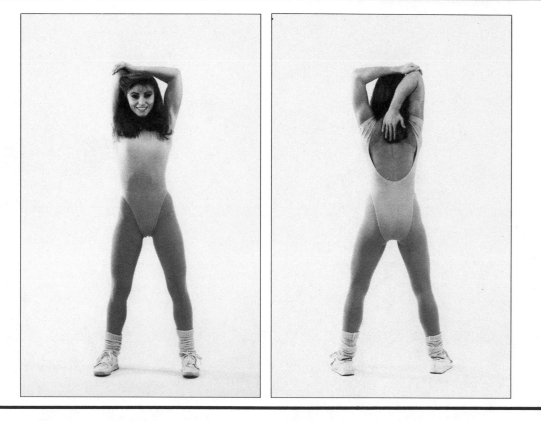

BACK OF ARM STRETCH: Basic standing position. Keeping the back straight and the shoulders relaxed down, bend the elbows above your head and place the left hand on the right elbow. (This stretch can also be done in the basic sitting position.)

With the left palm, press the right elbow down toward the center of your back. Feel the stretch in the back of your upper arm. Hold for eight to ten counts and release. Repeat the stretch with the left arm.

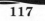

THE RUBBER BAND WORKOUTS

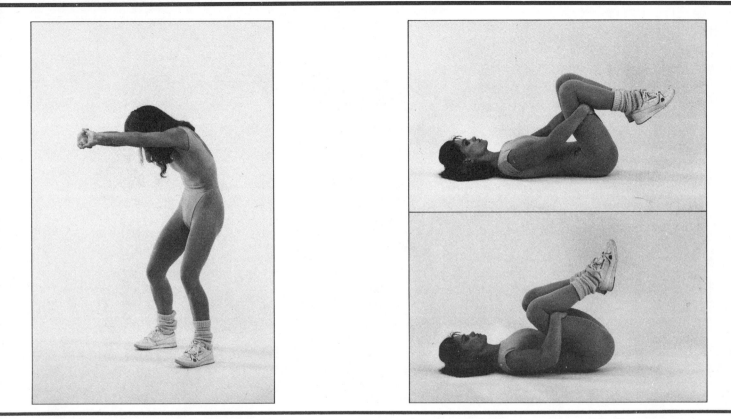

UPPER BACK STRETCH: Basic standing position with fingers laced and palms facing away from the body. Bend the knees, round the back and *press* the arms away from the body. Hold for eight to ten counts and release.

LOWER BACK STRETCH: Basic supine position with knees bent to hip level and hands held under the knees *(top)*. Pull the knees in toward the chest and try to touch the knees to the chest as you hold for eight to ten counts *(bottom)* and release.

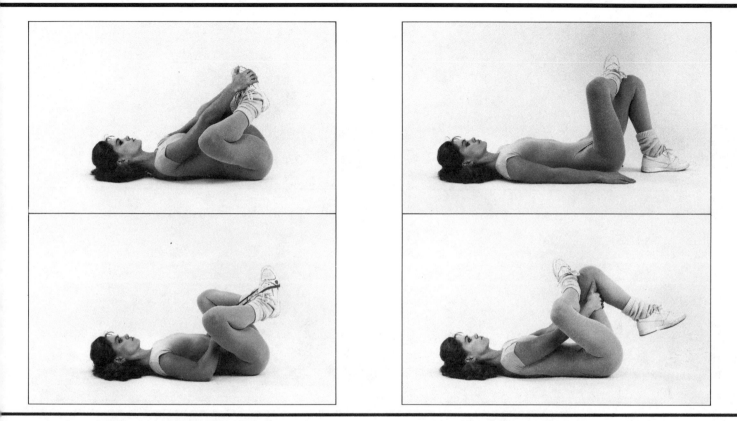

INNER THIGH STRETCH: Basic supine position. Bend the knees with the soles of the feet together. Open the thighs and place one end of the band around the feet or hold the feet with both hands *(top)*. Draw the feet in towards the center of the body, feeling the stretch in the inner thighs *(bottom)*. Hold for eight to ten counts and release.

OUTER THIGH STRETCH: Basic supine position. Cross your right ankle over your left knee *(top)*. Place the hands on the back of the left thigh and gently pull the left knee in toward the chest *(bottom)*. Hold for eight to ten counts and repeat the stretch on the other side.

THE RUBBER BAND WORKOUTS

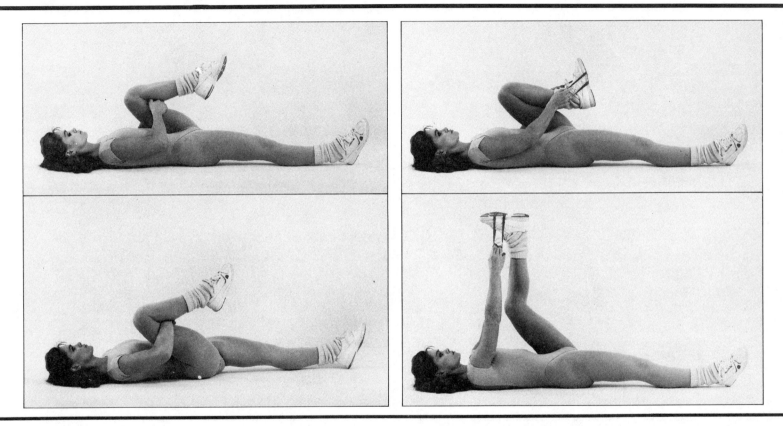

HIP FLEXOR STRETCH: Basic supine position. Hold the left knee in as close to the chest as possible and extend the right leg out straight, down to the floor. Press the back of the right knee to the floor. Feel the stretch in between the front of the thigh and the hip bone. Hold for eight to ten counts *(top)* and release. Repeat the stretch with the other leg.

BACK OF THIGH STRETCH: Basic supine position. Hold the double or single band at the ends, in fist grips. Keeping the right leg straight on the floor, bring the left knee in toward your chest and place the sole of the left foot on the band, fists on either side of the foot *(top)*. Extend the left leg, only to the point of tightness, not to pain *(bottom)*. Hold for eight to ten counts and release. Repeat the stretch with the right leg.

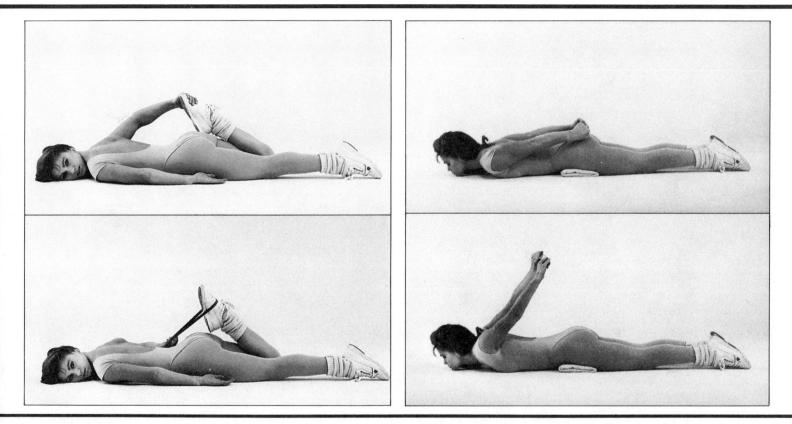

FRONT OF THIGH STRETCH: Basic prone position, with a towel under the hips, *(top)*. Use the band if you need it as an extension. With (or without) the band around the right foot, draw the right heel in toward the buttocks *(bottom)*. Feel the stretch in the front of the thighs. Hold for eight to ten counts and release. Repeat the stretch with the left leg. (This stretch can also be done in the basic standing position.)

SHOULDER AND CHEST STRETCH: Basic prone position, holding the single band in a fist grip behind your back *(top)*. (You can also do this stretch without the band.) Lift the arms up as high as they can comfortably go. Feel the stretch from your wrists to your arms to your shoulders to your chest *(bottom)*. Hold for eight to ten counts and release. (This stretch can also be done in the basic standing position.)

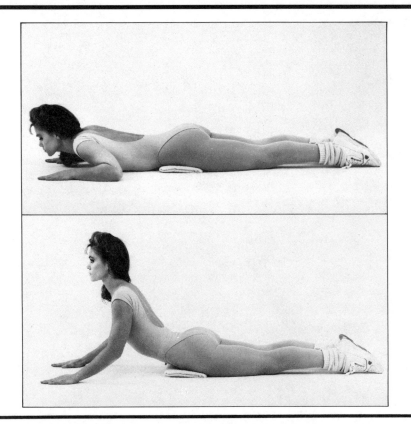

ABDOMINAL STRETCH: Basic prone position. Place the hands underneath the shoulders, elbows bent *(top)*. Keeping the hips on the floor, lift the upper body to the point of tightness, not to pain *(bottom)*. Feel the stretch in the abdominals. Hold for two to four counts (no more) and release down.

The Get-in-Shape Workout

It's never too late to get in shape. Once you have become familiar with the resistance exercises in Part Two, you can begin this program, which features one exercise for each muscle group. Use the beginning positions and the double band for the exercises until you see results or feel you are ready for more of a challenge. Then move on to the Stay-in-Shape Workout.

WARM-UP (3 to 5 minutes) to raise the body temperature and lubricate the joints;

STRETCHES (5 to 8 minutes) to increase muscle flexibility (optional here, essential after the workout);

AEROBICS (15 to 20 minutes of uninterrupted movement) to burn fat;

COOL-DOWN (3 to 5 minutes) to bring the heart rate down to normal after aerobics;

THE RUBBER BAND WORKOUT (10 to 15 minutes) to strengthen muscles;

STRETCHES (5 to 8 minutes) to increase muscle flexibility.

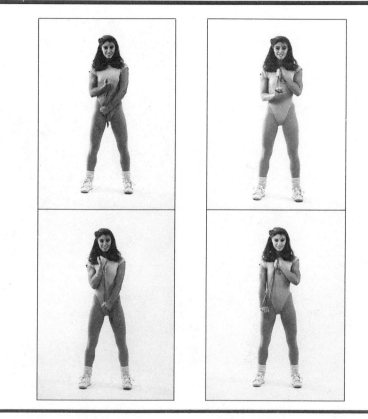

Front of Arm Curl
Repetitions: 8 to 12
  for each arm
Review: see page 36

*Back of Arm
Press-Down*
Repetitions: 8 to 12
  for each arm
Review: see page 42

THE RUBBER BAND WORKOUTS

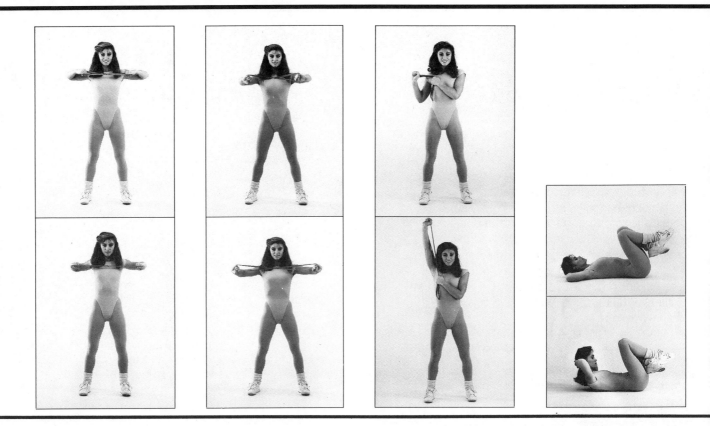

**Upper Back
  Conditioner**
Repetitions: 8 to 12
Review: see page 50

**All-Around Chest
  Conditioner**
Repetitions: 8 to 12
Review: see page 60

Shoulder Press-Up
Repetitions: 8 to 12
  for each arm
Review: see page 64

**Beginner Abdominal
  Curl, Without the
  Band**
Repetitions: 8 to 12
Review: see page 72

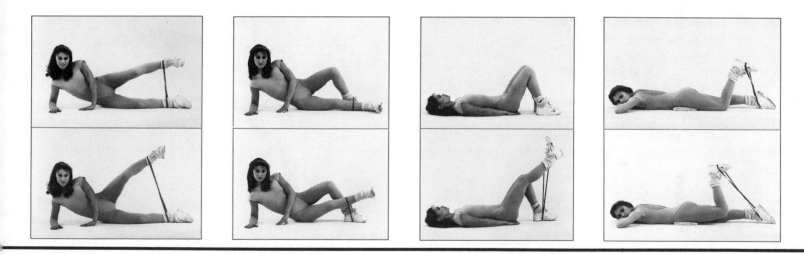

Outer Thigh Lift
Repetitions: 8 to 12 for
  each leg
Review: see page 78

Inner Thigh Lift
Repetitions: 8 to 12 for
  each leg
Review: see page 86

Front of Thigh Extension
Repetitions: 8 to 12 for
  each leg
Review: see page 90

Back of Thigh Lift
Repetitions: 8 to 12 for
  each leg
Review: see page 100

The Stay-in-Shape Workout

When you have done the Get-in-Shape Workout for about four weeks, and you feel you are strong enough, you are ready for the maintenance program. The elements are the same as the Get-in-Shape Workout, but the workout increases to two exercises per muscle group and uses the single rubber band.

Do this program no less than three days a week, alternating days.

WARM-UP (3 to 5 minutes) to raise the body temperature and lubricate the joints;

STRETCHES (5 to 8 minutes) to increase muscle flexibility
(optional here, essential after the workout);

AEROBICS (15 to 20 minutes of uninterrupted movement) to burn fat;

COOL-DOWN (3 to 5 minutes) to bring the heart rate down to normal after aerobics;

THE RUBBER BAND WORKOUT (10 to 15 minutes) to strengthen muscles;

STRETCHES (5 to 8 minutes) to increase muscle flexibility.

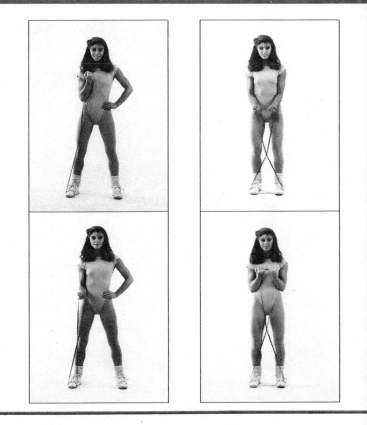

Front of Arm Curl with Foot
Repetitions: 12 to 16 for each arm
Review: see page 38

Double-Arm Curl
Repetitions: 12 to 16
Review: see page 40

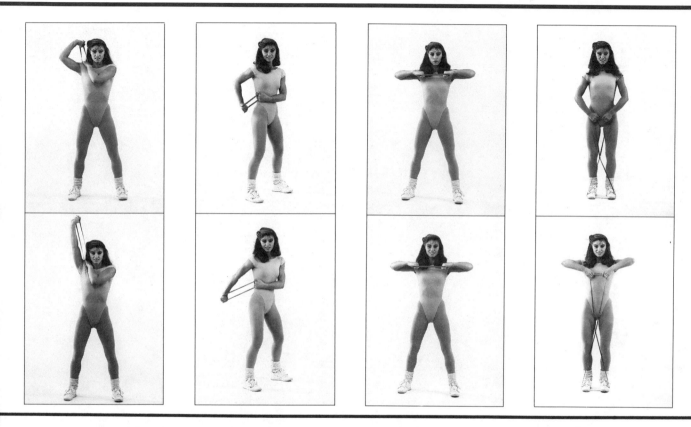

Back of Arm Press-Up
Repetitions: 12 to 16
  for each arm
Review: see page 46

**Back of Arm
  Press-Back**
Repetitions: 12 to 16
  for each arm
Review: see page 48

**Upper Back
  Conditioner**
Repetitions: 12 to 16
Review: see page 50

Upright Row
Repetitions: 12 to 16
Review: see page 56

THE RUBBER BAND WORKOUTS

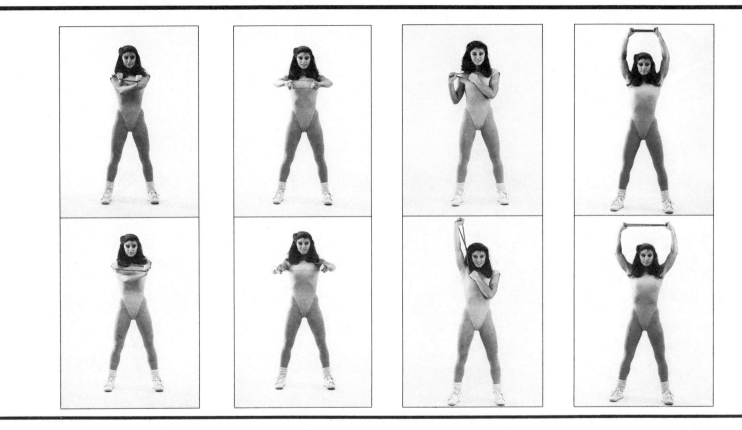

Chest Crossover
Repetitions: 12 to 16
Review: see page 58

All-Around Chest Conditioner
Repetitions: 12 to 16
Review: see page 60

Shoulder Press-Up
Repetitions: 12 to 16
  for each arm
Review: see page 64

Shoulder Press-Out
Repetitions: 12 to 16
Review: see page 68

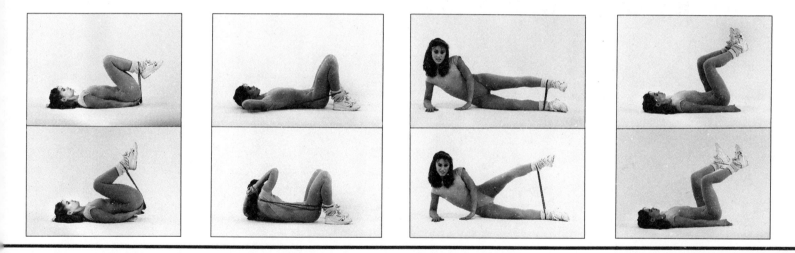

Advanced Reverse Abdominal Curl with the Band
Repetitions: 12 to 16
Review: see page 74

Abdominal Crossover
Repetitions: 12 to 16 on each side
Review: see page 76

Outer Thigh Lift
Repetitions: 12 to 16 for each leg
Review: see page 78

Outer Thigh Press-Out
Repetitions: 12 to 16
Review: see page 82

THE RUBBER BAND WORKOUTS

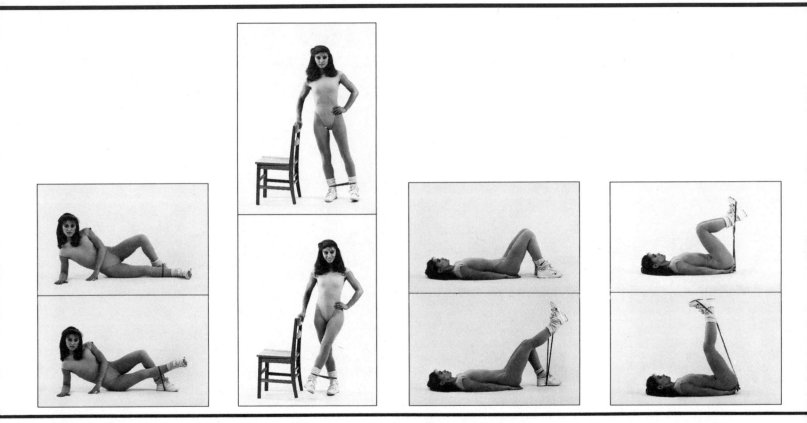

Inner Thigh Lift
Repetitions: 12 to 16
  for each leg
Review: see page 86

**Inner Thigh Lift,
Standing**
Repetitions: 12 to 16
  for each leg
Review: see page 88

Front of Thigh Extension
Repetitions: 12 to 16 for
  each leg
Review: see page 90

Two-Leg Extension
Repetitions: 12 to 16
Review: see page 94

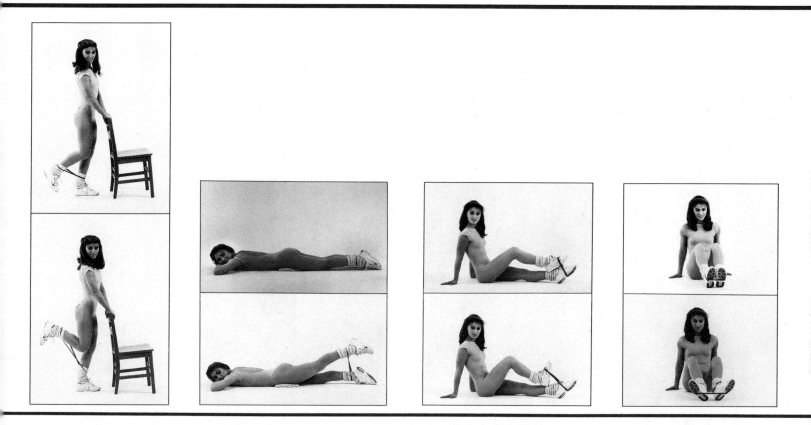

Back of Thigh Curl, Standing
Repetitions: 12 to 16 for each leg
Review: see page 98

Straight-Leg Lift
Repetitions: 12 to 16 for each leg
Review: see page 102

Shin Strengthener
Repetitions: 8 to 12 for each leg
Review: see page 106

Shin Strengthener, Variation
Repetitions: 8 to 12 for each leg
Review: see page 107

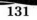

The Chair Workout

When you can't get to your complete program, when you are sitting at your desk or watching television, or when you are ready to try something different, do the Chair Workout. The beginner would use the double band; the advanced, the single band.

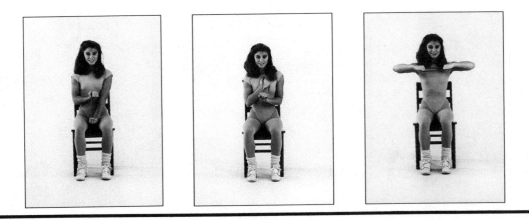

Front of Arm Curl
Repetitions: 12 to 16
for each arm
Review: see page 36

Back of Arm
Press-Down
Repetitions: 12 to 16
for each arm
Review: see page 42

Upper Back
Conditioner
Repetitions: 12 to 16
Review: see page 50

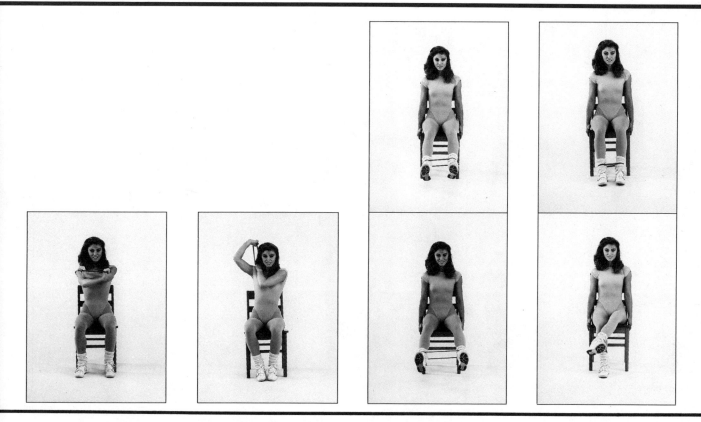

Chest Crossover
Repetitions: 12 to 16
Review: see page 58

Shoulder Press-Up
Repetitions: 12 to 16
Review: see page 64

Outer Thigh Press-Out, Seated
Repetitions: 12 to 16
Review: see page 84

Inner Thigh Lift, Seated
Repetitions: 12 to 16
   for each leg
Review: see page 88

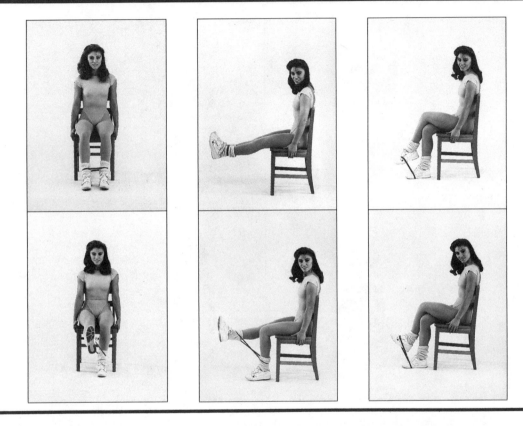

Front of Thigh Extension, Variation
Repetitions: 12 to 16 for each leg
Review: see page 93

Back of Thigh Curl, Seated
Repetitions: 12 to 16 for each leg
Review: see page 99

Shin Strengthener
Repetitions: 8 to 12 for each leg
Review: see page 106

The Ten-Minute Workout

There is no longer any excuse for not exercising. This workout is designed for the busy person on the go or for when the longer program doesn't fit that day's schedule.

Carry the band with you in your briefcase or purse. When you have ten minutes, pull it out and do one exercise per muscle group. Save the warm-up, stretches, and aerobics for when you have more time.

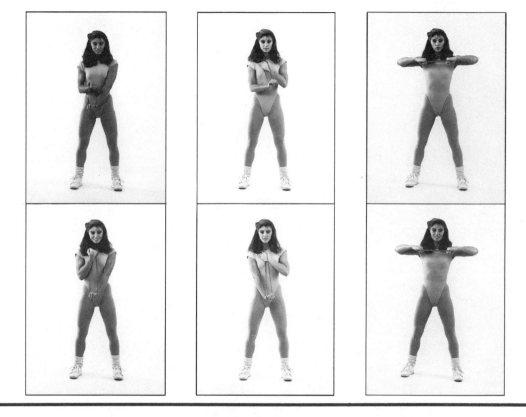

Front of Arm Curl
Repetitions: 12 to 16
  for each arm
Review: see page 36

Back of Arm Press-Down
Repetitions: 12 to 16
  for each arm
Review: see page 42

Upper Back Conditioner
Repetitions: 12 to 16
Review: see page 50

THE RUBBER BAND WORKOUTS

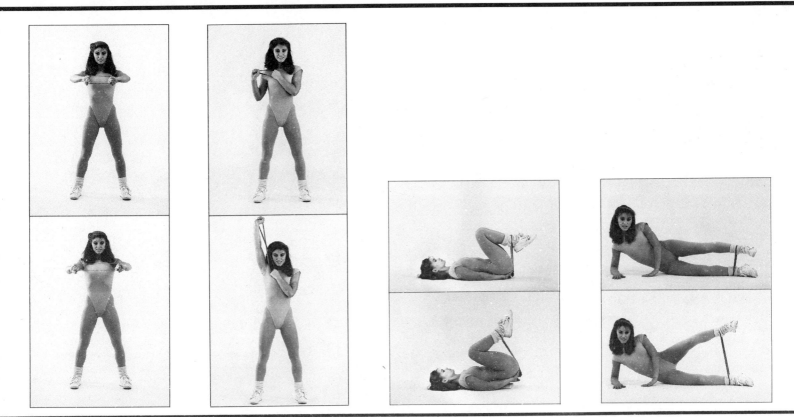

**All-Around Chest
Conditioner**
Repetitions: 12 to 16
Review: see page 60

Shoulder Press-Ups
Repetitions: 12 to 16
for each arm
Review: see page 64

**Advanced Reverse
Abdominal Curl,
with the Band**
Repetitions: 12 to 16
Review: see page 74

Outer Thigh Lift
Repetitions: 12 to 16
for each leg
Review: see page 78

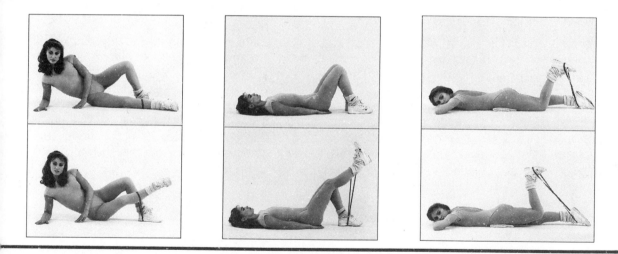

Inner Thigh Lift
Repetitions: 12 to 16
  for each leg
Review: see page 86

**_Front of Thigh
  Extension_**
Repetitions: 12 to 16
  for each leg
Review: see page 90

**_Back of Thigh Curl,
  Prone Position_**
Repetitions: 12 to 16
  for each leg
Review: see page 96

The Power Workout

This is the challenge workout, the very advanced program for the well-conditioned individual. Be realistic about whether you're really ready for this. And if you feel any pain or discomfort in the joints when you do the resistance exercises, stop at once.

You can use the two *single* ⅝-inch rubber bands that came with this book as if they were one band or order thicker bands from SPRI Products (see page 139). I use the 1-inch band for the upper body and the 1½-inch band for the lower body and I highly recommend them. Although using the two single bands together does work, I think it's a lot easier to use one thicker one.

The Power Workout is flexible, but it is important that you work each muscle or muscle group. You can follow the selection of exercises in the Get-in-Shape Workout, or you can put together your own sequence, as long as you include at least one for each muscle group. Do 12 to 16 repetitions of each exercise and do the complete workout three times.

You can choose to do 12 to 16 repetitions of each exercise in your routine, and then repeat the complete workout sequence two more times. Or you can do three groups of 12 to 16 repetitions of one exercise *before* proceeding on to the next exercise. But if you choose this alternative, you must rest between each set of repetitions for about one minute, so that the muscles can relax.

WARM-UP (3 to 5 minutes) to raise the body temperature and lubricate the joints;

STRETCHES (8 to 10 minutes) to increase muscle flexibility (optional here, essential after the workout);

AEROBICS (20 to 30 minutes of uninterrupted movement) to burn fat;

COOL-DOWN (3 to 5 minutes) to bring the heart rate down to normal after aerobics;

THE RUBBER BAND WORKOUT (20 minutes) to strengthen muscles;

STRETCHES (10 minutes) to increase muscle flexibility.

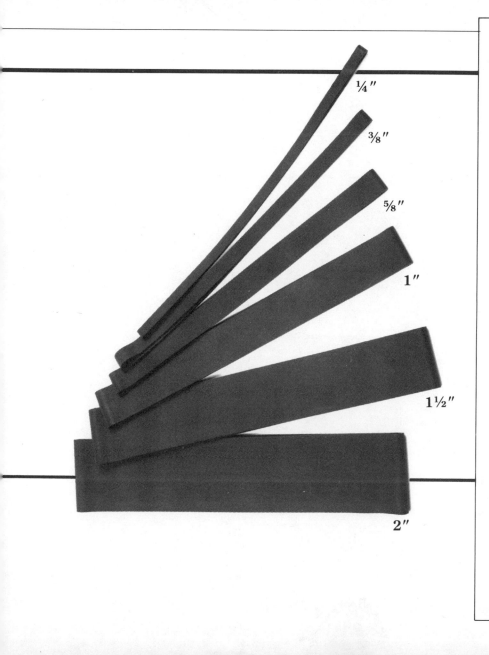

¼"

⅜"

⅝"

1"

1½"

2"

Tamilee Webb's Original Rubber Band Workout
comes with two ⅝" bands. To purchase additional bands, or bands of other widths, use this order form.

☐ Please send me the following SPRI (Sports Performance & Rehabilitation Institute) bands:

_____	¼" wide @	$_____	= _____
_____	⅜" wide @	_____	= _____
_____	⅝" wide @	_____	= _____
_____	1" wide @	_____	= _____
_____	1½" wide @	_____	= _____
_____	2" wide @	_____	= _____

SUBTOTAL _____
+ SHIPPING & HANDLING _____
+ ILLINOIS RESIDENTS
ADD 7% SALES TAX _____
TOTAL _____

SPRI BAND PRICES PER BAND

QUANTITY	¼" WIDE	⅜" WIDE	⅝" WIDE	1" WIDE	1½" WIDE	2" WIDE
1–9	$1.00	$1.25	$1.75	$2.50	$3.25	$4.00
10–49	.50	.60	.80	1.00	1.40	2.00
50–99	.40	.50	.70	.80	1.20	1.70
100–249	.35	.45	.60	.70	1.10	1.60
250–499	.30	.40	.50	.60	1.00	1.50
500–999	.25	.35	.45	.55	.95	1.45

SHIPPING & HANDLING CHARGES

FOR ORDERS OF	ADD	FOR ORDERS OF	ADD
Up to $10	$1.75	$35.01 to $50	$5.00
$10.01 to $25	$3.00	$50.01 to $75	$6.25
$25.01 to $35	$4.00	$75.01 to $100	$8.00

Name _____

Company or Organization _____

Street Address _____

City _____ State _____ Zip _____

Mail check or money order to:
SPRI Products, Inc.
962 N. Northwest Hwy.
Park Ridge, IL 60068

Or telephone:
Inside Illinois call:
312–823–0090
Outside Illinois call Toll Free:
1–800–222–7774